Anne Diamond

A NEW YOU

Start Your New Life Today

First published 2003 by Contender Books
Contender Books is a division of
The Contender Entertainment Group
48 Margaret Street
London W1W 8SE
www.contenderbooks.com

This edition published 2003

1 3 5 7 9 10 8 6 4 2

Text © Anne Diamond

ISBN 1 84357 107 2

Cover and text design by Button One-to-One
Typesetting by E-Type
Repro by Radstock Reproductions, Midsomer Norton, Bath
Printed and bound in the UK by Butler & Tanner Ltd, Frome and London
Production by Kate Gribble

Plate section photographs supplied by Anne Diamond, Channel 4, Universal
Pictorial Press, Mark Richards and the *Daily Mail*, Alan Olley and Scope Features.
New photography by Phil Surbey.
Cover photography by Phil Surbey and Rex Features.
Kind thanks go to Marks and Spencer for their contribution to this book.

**Before starting any weight loss plan, it is highly advisable to consult your GP.
This plan is not recommended whilst you are pregnant, breastfeeding or have
an active medical condition.**

Anne Diamond

A NEW YOU

Start Your New Life Today

contents

chapter 1

life in the fat lane

When I think about it – and if I am really honest – I have always had a 'thing' about my weight. I don't remember it being an issue when I was little, but by the time I went to senior school, and mini skirts were all the rage, I had become conscious of the fact that my legs simply weren't up to the task that the sixties had set them.

Everyone else seemed to have perfect legs – and even those girls in my class who were a bit gawky, owned legs they could show off without fear of denigration. My legs fell into the plump variety – and at only five feet and four inches, I was never going to grow tall enough for them to even out on their own.

Again, though (and thank goodness, really), it was never a huge issue amongst us schoolgirls. Maybe it was because mini skirts were the fashion must-have of the time, and you couldn't opt out of that rule – *everybody* wore them – that you were never pointed out.

Girls far larger than I wore minis and proudly showed off the top of their 'hold-up' tights, too! (Miss Harvey and Miss Jeffries regularly held mini skirt sessions where we girls would have to kneel down on the floor, and they would hold a big ruler up to our knees, to test the height of our skirts. Of course, as soon as that was over, we would roll over the waistband several times so that our skirts became pelmets again!) When I think of it, we strapping lasses were a testament to British beef at its best. Or maybe we were the first mad cows? Whatever, none of us had hang-ups about our size – it was just a fact of life.

I do remember, though, being very embarrassed about my elephantine legs when the photographs came back from my sister's wedding. I must have been seventeen at the time. You would never look at *that* girl, with those massive thighs in that micro mini skirt, and predict 'she is going to have a big career in television'! You'd be more likely to think I might make a successful career in the haulage business.

Some scientists reckon you develop your tendency to a weight problem from very early life – maybe even as far back as in the womb. So you can wave an accusing finger at your mother. What did she eat during your pregnancy? Did she wean you too soon, and on to the wrong sorts of foods?

I know my mother always remembers that she used to put an extra spoonful of formula into my bottle of milk. It was 1954 and, as it was post war – and rationing had only just been phased out – she says it was a matter of pride to many mothers that they should have a 'bonny baby'. It was almost a competition every week, to see whose baby had put on the most weight. You were the talk of the baby clinic if your child was skinny, or undernourished – so many mothers fed their babies up, like turkeys for Christmas. My mum says she was always very proud of my sturdy legs. Mmmm. That was all very well in 1954. Trouble is, I've still got them!

Still, you cannot start blaming mum, can you? We are all free to make our own choices, and anyway, my weight has never been a constant, big or small. If I look back through the picture albums, I go from little to large in a matter of months – and as soon as mini skirts went out of fashion, I hid my legs behind midis or maxis and now – permanently – trousers. But there's one fashion item that has always bugged me: knee-high boots. I have never been able to zip the darn things all the way up. I have always hated shopping for boots – because they're still the one item that can instantly bring back all the awfulness of those awkward teenage years, when I felt hopelessly inadequate and sometimes quite despairing of my legs.

How I ever summoned up the courage to appear in a bikini in an amateur drama in my home town, I will never know. I was offered one of the leading roles in a comedy called 'The Man Most Likely To' – a great part. Only when I had accepted it, and was into the second reading, did I realise that it was essential that my character flounce around in a bikini in act two! Dreading that moment nearly spoiled the entire play for me. One thing was for sure. Funny how I have not kept one photograph from that play!

Starting work seemed to slim me down a lot – maybe because I was too busy to think much about my weight – or maybe (and more likely) it was because I was living a hectic lifestyle where I was always dashing around, and possibly only ever ate one decent meal a day. Whatever the truth, it is interesting to remember in view of the fact that my recent war on weight has coincided with my leaving full-time TV work and taking up writing!

I was at a dinner party recently with friends I hadn't seen for about twenty years. They said they were astounded to see me on *Big Brother*, and even more amazed to see how I had ballooned in weight.

'When you were on *TV-am*, you were always *so tiny*!' they chirped.

And yet, while I was sitting on that golden sofa for nearly eight years, I was never once happy with my weight, my shape. I always felt body conscious, always inadequate...

I remember being so envious of Wincey Willis, our weather girl. We often went out to fashion shops, and met the designers, together. She could try anything on, and immediately look good. She was a couple of inches taller than me – and very svelte. I was bulgy, and the bulges always seemed to be in the wrong places. I had to struggle to find anything that looked right on me – it used to make me so sick!

During those years, I did consciously diet once. It was when I was asked to present Miss World. It was 1985, the first year that the organisers, Julia and Ken Morley, had decided to go without their regular presenter, Judith Chalmers, and try someone else.

They had probably thought (and I wince to think of it now) that their lady presenter should be younger, slimmer and more gorgeous. I remember how the newspapers jibed at Judith Chalmers at the time. Someone very unkind in one tabloid (and look how it has stuck in my memory) said that Ms Chalmers at the last Miss World had worn a white dress which made her look like a big fridge on stage. I wonder if Judith Chalmers saw what they wrote about me when I left *Big Brother*…?

It was a great compliment to be asked to present Miss World, but I knew that – quite literally – the world would be watching me. Yet who was I to *stand with* on stage, at no less a venue than the Royal Albert Hall – in front of an estimated 18 million viewers?

Twenty of the most beautiful girls in the entire world – all perfect, pert breasts and long silky legs, plus the long, lithe and elegant Mrs Morley, that's who!

I was already a trim size 10/12 – but, knowing that TV cameras are notorious for putting at least half a stone on you, I concluded that I had better starve myself into a size 8.

It was great! One of Princess Diana's most trusted and talented designers, Bruce Oldfield, was to make my dress. Knowing I would be seen a lot from behind (as I was interviewing the girls about how they all aspired to be brain surgeons), Bruce designed a big diamond-shaped cut-out on my back. The fabric was a dark, shimmering silk velvet.

Every week, I went along for a fitting – and every week, they had to make adjustments because I had lost so much weight. I was positively petite by the time of the show.

The Royal Albert Hall is a pretty awesome place, when you are on the stage in the centre of the spotlight, and there are hundreds in the audience, and millions watching you on TV. I felt like a million dollars, though, because I was confident of how I looked.

I cannot even remember who won the contest that night. It didn't matter. I was on a high. It was the first night in my whole life, I think, that I was entirely happy with my body. We went out for a celebratory dinner afterwards, and I ate for Britain.

That was also the last time I was ever a size 8!

I haven't been able to get that dress on since. It's still upstairs, in the wardrobe, waiting…

From that moment onwards, it was yo-yo land for me. Up and down, highs and lows – my weight careered from one month to the next like a car on a switchback ride. I would try one diet, and then another. Most of them were ridiculous, all of them were torture. Some helped a little, by banning one sort of food, or encouraging weird combinations. I could stick at them for a while, summoning all my will power, depriving myself of the foods I fancied, and moaning about it to anyone within hearing distance. And then, months later, I would notice that my clothes were getting tight again.

Of course, five pregnancies didn't help. I managed to keep my weight under control during my first pregnancy – and still looked pretty slim in the mother and baby photographs. But when I was expecting my

11

second son, James, we went to Australia during the last few months of my pregnancy, and I compensated for the hot weather by drinking gallons of fizzy orange and eating a thousand ice creams (Walls made one in Oz called 'Gaytime'. Oh, it was my favourite! I wonder if they still have them – and whether they've at last changed the name?!).

After Jamie was born, I had to find a trainer to come to my house to help me work off the excess two stones. I mistakenly thought I could never, ever put on so much weight again. I blamed Australia for having no calorie-free drinks.

My trainer was called Clayton. He was brilliant, because once you had made an appointment with him, he was unstoppable. If I woke up one day and decided bed was too tempting to leave, I would give him a call.

'You cannot put me off, I'm coming around anyway!' he would laugh. He meant it. He would storm into the house, make straight for the kitchen, fling open the fridge door and shout: 'What are these sausages doing in here?'

'They're for the kids, honest!' I would splutter.

'They'd better be!' he would grunt, and then give me a lecture about sausages.

I hate to tell you this if you are a sausage lover – but once you know exactly what's in the things, you won't want them any more, I promise you. I have never touched one since.

That taught me a lesson, too! That you can give up certain foods if you can convince yourself – deep inside your brain – that you really don't fancy them any more, whatever the reason.

Once I learned what was in the average sausage (gristle, fat, minced offal – the list goes on and gets more disgusting), I just couldn't face eating them any more. For fifteen years, I haven't eaten a sausage. I have never required will power to resist them and I haven't once felt deprived. I still like the smell of them sizzling in the pan – but I just cannot eat one.

Now, if my brain can switch my likes and dislikes so strongly and so effectively over one type of food – so that I don't even need will power to make the change – then surely it can do the same with other foods?

I wish I had stopped then and there and thought harder about it – because it might have prevented the following decade of dieting misery and despair that, despite a hectic and hugely successful career in the media spotlight, it was my body that was always letting me down.

No one understands unless they've been there themselves. When you feel really unhappy about your body image, you do crazy things. You say no to invitations you've always dreamed of. You dread being asked out to dinner. You hate shopping for clothes, and loathe trying things on. You can't relax when you're naked – even in your own home. And what about sex? You dread the thought of meeting someone nice, because he will have to (at some point) see your body. Some women even stay with horrible husbands because their body image is so low, they feel they must be unattractive to anyone else. You get that horrid feeling in the pit of your stomach when someone gets out the camera and asks for a picture! (Can you imagine how many times that has happened to me?) You always hide behind others for photos, or offer to take the picture of everyone else. You hate holidays, because you know you are going to have to make an exhibition of yourself on a beach. Your kids beg you to come swimming with them, and instead you stay sweltering on the poolside under a large floppy hat, sunspecs and the biggest sarong the beach boutique could offer. I have even turned down personal appearances and TV work because I felt my body would let me down.

So when *Big Brother* asked me to appear on their second 'Celebrity' show, I naturally said no. Quite firmly. Far too exposing!

I'd never actually seen *Big Brother*. Obviously, I'd caught snippets while channel-hopping and I was aware of all the hype – the fact that it wove some sort of strange black magic which turned monosyllabic kids who'd never done a day's training into stars who were suddenly worth their own chat show. But I had also heard about the first celebrity version – where people had apparently gone quite mad.

Not me, I said. Not *Big Brother*, no way! No – no way – not me. That's for beautiful bodies like Anthea Turner and er… Vanessa Feltz.

Then my children started nagging.

It would be so cool, they said. In the end, I bent under the pressure, and to my horror – almost as though I was having an out-of-body experience – I found myself actually sitting in front of the *Big Brother* production team, saying, OK, yes, I'll do it.

(There's no money in it whatsoever, by the way, so you really do have to be mad…)

Mind you, that's when all the papers were saying that Graham Norton and Dawn French had already agreed to do it. I thought, if they're daft enough to risk their careers, then who am I to say no?

A week after I'd agreed, they gave me the final list – and Dawn French and Graham Norton were nowhere on it. Instead, Melinda Messenger and Les Dennis, Mark Owen, Sue Perkins (from Mel and Sue) and Goldie, the film actor and 'garage' DJ were to be my fellow housemates.

Only then did I think – if there's no Dawn French, then I am definitely going to be the largest lady in town. And the press will make mincemeat of me. After all, I'd always been known as the elfin Queen of Breakfast Television. What would they make of me now I had mysteriously put on about five stones?

I rang around all my friends – particularly those who knew the media and its moods.

Don't worry, they said, each and every one of them. No one will dare criticise you too much for your weight. It would be so non PC, so insulting to so many of their female readers. After all, 46% of women in the UK are size 16 plus… They might have a little dig – but it can't go any further.

Well, well! How wrong we all were.

No sooner had I clambered up that giant metal staircase to the *Big Brother* house, and clonked my metal suitcase up behind me, than the Grande Dames of Fleet Street had their knives out, their sharpened talons poised at their word processors.

Lynda Lee Potter must have thought Christmas had come early. My carcass had fallen neatly on to her butcher's block. I was positively begging for a dressing down. She hanged, drew and quartered me, and then stuck my remains on the spikes of her Wednesday column. Anne Diamond's children must be ashamed, she said, to have a mother with such a gargantuan bottom.

And under a headline which read – on the front page – 'she's sad, lonely and desperate', a male reporter wrote 'whatever happened to her youth and beauty? She's a middle-aged mum without a man…'

Luckily, cooped up inside the mirrored madhouse, I couldn't read it. Indeed, we weren't allowed to take in anything to read. Researchers even went through everything – and I mean every sock, shoe and slipper inside my suitcase – to make sure I hadn't smuggled in any pens or pencils or anything at all that could be used as a writing implement. They even confiscated my eyebrow pencil!

By the time I was evicted – after a week in there which felt like a year

– the press had got over my change in shape, and instead wanted to know the inside story of Les Dennis, his surreal relationship with the *Big Brother* chickens and the beginning of his marital nightmare.

Thanks, Les, for taking the spotlight off my gargantuan behind.

When I finally read the newspaper cuttings, I simply couldn't believe it.

Clearly my excess weight spelled out the end of a meaningful life for me. By putting on a few stones, and then having the sheer nerve to display myself on national television, I had signalled my fall to the depths of shamelessness and degeneracy.

Worse than an alcoholic who had been found lying in the gutter, a serial adulterer caught leaving a seedy back-street brothel, or even a celebrity junkie snapped snorting cocaine, I had been exposed as a woman who had 'Let Herself Go'. Implicit in all the nasty comments was a moral judgement – it wasn't that I had simply put on weight, I must have lost control of my life, thrown away my values, abandoned all principle and gone to the dogs.

Indeed, because I had joked (several times and with jolly good reason!) in the *Big Brother* house that I would love a drink, the press decided I was an alcoholic, too. That just completed the tawdry picture.

I was truly shocked that any writer could pen the sort of vitriol that was hurled my way – and solely because I was fat.

All right – so that is in itself a naive comment. Of course, the British press often enjoys being downright abusive. Sometimes, certain papers deliberately set out to hound celebrities, making their lives pretty miserable. But to make moral judgements and malign any woman for simply putting on weight? Well, that really is tantamount to insulting so many of their readers. You wouldn't dare say that on TV, I can tell you. Because you know just what your viewers would do about it. They'd switch off, that's what they'd do.

Still in shock, I remember driving the kids to school just a couple of days after I had been released from the *Big Brother* house. I was listening to my local radio station, Fox FM. They were talking about a particularly nasty piece about me in that morning's *Daily Mail*.

'I think this is absolutely appalling,' said one of the morning DJs. 'They have said some really dreadful things about Anne Diamond – and just because she's put on a bit of weight.'

Several listeners phoned in, agreeing.

'I tell you what, why don't we all boycott that newspaper?' suggested one. 'If that's how they feel about fat ladies, then let's show them what we think about their paper!'

Is this shameful attitude towards fatties just the fault of our opinionated media? I don't think so – it may be a British thing. Just compare us to others in Europe or America.

In France, well, a woman just wouldn't get fat, and that's all there is to it. There must be fat Frenchwomen somewhere, mustn't there? But you never see them... In nearly every other European country, a fat momma is a sign of security, motherly warmth, great cooking and down-to-earth values!

You only have to pop over the pond to Florida to find that the fattest people in the world are not ashamed of their size. Heck, they waddle around in shorts and bikini tops you could camp overnight in. If you want a real holiday, I recommend DisneyWorld, Universal Studios, Busch Gardens and SeaWorld. Not just because they are fantastic places for a family vacation, but because you'll always feel so minuscule compared to the vast majority of the women there!

We could do with a little more of that tolerance here – that body confidence. Instead, we Brits hide ourselves away – ashamed to go out, frightened to be seen eating, lest we attract criticism for 'Letting Ourselves Go'.

Not that I am saying fat is good. It isn't. It is unhealthy to be obese – and we in Britain are facing an obesity epidemic. If you're 5' 5'' and you're over eleven stones, you are clinically obese.

I am sorry if that hurts. Unfortunately it is true. And obesity means you could be facing Type 2 diabetes, problems with your blood pressure, strokes, heart disease, joint pains and all sorts of other concerns. If you are not suffering now, then you are storing up problems for the future.

I hate the word 'obese' – it sounds dirty, somehow! But I fell into that category myself – just a year ago. Then I looked at my kids and thought: what kind of example am I to them? And don't I want to do everything in my power to try to ensure that I am with them for as long as I possibly can be? So I don't just owe it to myself to be healthy – I owe it to them!

Many large ladies might feel I am letting them down by trying to lose weight – because I am definitely not waving the flag of liberation for fatties everywhere. I am not shouting to the rooftops: 'I am proud to be fat!'

On the contrary, I think it is a big mistake to be overweight. Sorry if you think I have sold out. But the truth is, I hate being fat and I hate being unfit – and I was both. Some women may actually like being big, although I seriously doubt it. I think if you could offer any of them the chance to lose all their excess fat with the simple wave of a wand, then they would jump at the opportunity. The problem is that there is no easy or instant solution.

I think many women fool themselves they like being fat – it's a defensive reaction to all the jibes, unkind comments and criticism like I experienced. Other fat ladies may have tried and tried, diet after diet, and ended up resigning themselves to life in the fat lane.

I know how hard it is and can quite understand why. Indeed, if it hadn't been for the harsh words of those appalling writers after the *Big Brother* experience, I might be still there, in my extra-large T-shirt and baggy trousers, trying and failing on another diet.

But this time, I made it.

I found a different way. I threw away the diet books and the calorie calculators – and I started eating really, really well.

QUIZ: Are you ruled by negative feelings about your looks?

Just one year ago, I did a quiz rather like this one, and found that I was becoming obsessed with my body image – and that it was preventing me from doing many exciting things. My feelings about my body were quite literally ruling my life. See how you score by putting yourself into a few everyday situations, and testing your reactions. Be honest now!

1. You are out and about – then you catch sight of your reflection in a mirror or shop window. DO YOU:

A: Smile at yourself and continue with what you were doing.

B: Suck your stomach in, and starve yourself the rest of the day.

C: Feel instantly depressed, go home and eat a whole packet of Hobnobs.

2. When you're trying on clothes in a shop changing room. DO YOU:

A: Wish you could buy the lot – they're all perfect!

B: Struggle to find something that will fit and look good.

C: Find nothing you like that'll fit, and leave in tears.

3. When you're on holiday, on the beach, or at the poolside. DO YOU:

A: Wear a bikini – if you've got it, flaunt it!

B: Carefully choose a one-piece and sarong that will cover all your bulges.

C: Cover up like it's winter, and avoid getting into the water.

4. When you're in the gym, or doing sport. DO YOU:

A: Wear the latest lycra gear – and strut your stuff confidently.

B: Choose a baggy T-shirt and leggings and leave before you get too sweaty.

C: You don't do anything physical – it's too embarrassing and uncomfortable.

5. When people see you before you've done yourself up. DO YOU:

A: Beam at them and tell them they have now seen you naked!

B: Pretend you are the cleaning lady and can you take a message for the boss?

C: Sniff a lot and croak that you are very ill.

6. When you're among a group of slimmer, good-looking women. DO YOU:

A: Enjoy the friendship of like-minded ladies.

B: Nip to the loo every ten minutes to check your make-up and dress.

C: Feel like the village frump, and resolve to make new, fat friends.

7. When you hear other women whispering and laughing. DO YOU:

A: Hardly notice them – you've got better things to do.

B: Automatically assume they are saying something catty about your body.

C: Run.

8. After you get a new haircut or hairstyle. DO YOU:

A: Go out to the next available social event to show it off.

B: Desperately hope it flatters your body shape.

C: I'll get a new hairdo when I've lost some weight.

9. When you've just met a new, attractive man, DO YOU:

A: Flirt outrageously and look forward to a steamy night.

B: Try to sound intelligent and hope he'll like your mind.

C: Tell him you're gay, then cry yourself to sleep alone.

10. When you're thinking about or having sex. DO YOU:

A: Concentrate on how his body looks, and forget about yours.

B: Insist you only get turned on in pitch darkness.

C: Sex? Don't you have to take your clothes off for that?

If your answers are...

Mostly As – then you are body confident, whatever your size. I admire you – I wish I was so self-assured and positive about life. That sort of confidence is immensely attractive to people. But do be honest with yourself. If you are overweight, then apply all that positive energy to healthier eating and a little more exercise.

Mostly Bs – you are beginning to lose confidence in yourself, because you sense you might be gaining weight – or maybe you have been trying to lose weight for a while, and you're despairing when diets let you down. Stop the rot now, before you become obsessed with your body shape and the way you see it. Life is there to be lived – don't say no to things just because you think you are too fat. Resolve to change your eating and exercise habits, starting today. You can enjoy life, WHILE you are changing your life*style*.

Mostly Cs – Aargh! You have fallen into the body-hating trap – and if you despise your body, then it's hard to get motivated. After all, why should you do it any favours? It's one thing to be a little self-conscious every now and then, and it's another thing entirely to be so consumed by insecurity that you can't enjoy making love. Stop letting bad feelings about flab keep you from feeling good! Remember that the real you IS inside that body – and you deserve better. You must learn to love yourself again – the you inside. Visualise how great things are going to be when you have changed your whole lifestyle, learned to love food again instead of seeing it as an enemy, learned to be part of the real world again. Start living again now – you deserve it!

chapter 2

a light at the end of the dieting tunnel

It all started when I met the Juice Master, a fresh-faced and very bushy-tailed (British!) guy called Jason Vale.

Now – don't be put off by the word 'juice'. I was put off by it for several months – and I lost valuable time when I could have been changing my life.

Friends said to me – have you met this guy, the Juice Master? He's lost tons of weight himself, and he might be able to make a difference with you.

I tut-tutted. I knew all about juicing. In my time, I have interviewed a hundred juice experts from the States. They tell you to buy cartloads of fruit. You come home from the supermarket laden down like a Covent Garden barrow boy, you bung it all into a juicing machine. You drink it. Then, about four days later, when the novelty has faded, you get fed up with it, shove it away in the back of a cupboard, then watch the fruit rot in the bottom of the fridge while you delve into a comforting mug of Pot Noodles.

I know all about it, I said.

I have been there, done it and got the T-shirt, I said. I can't be bothered with all that juice and pulp, peeling, coring, shopping and washing up.

I don't need to meet him.

My friends hung back. They know me well. Push me into doing something or meeting someone and I will resist as hard as I can, out of sheer stubbornness. I also cannot stand it if someone tries to advise me about my weight. If I am at a party, and about to grab a nacho with a huge dollop of salsa on it, and a friend says: 'Now – you shouldn't be eating that, should you?' – I will quite deliberately shove it in my mouth.

Is it to spite them, or merely to establish who's boss? Whatever the reason – unsolicited, helpful, well-meaning advice on the subject of my weight brings out the very worst in me. In fact, it makes me fatter!

So I steadfastly refused to meet Jason Vale, this juicing guru who, according to my friends, might change my life! I battled on with diets I read about in magazines, diets of the Hollywood stars (who, by the way, have *never ever* had a weight problem in their lives!), so-called revolutionary diets and oh, yes, of course, I had another go at the Atkins diet. (Absolutely hopeless for me, since I am a vegetarian and you need to eat your way through half a carcass of meat in the first week, as far as I can see!)

And still, I wasn't losing a pound.

In the end, I joined a slimming club, where the diet coach visits you in your home once or twice a week.

I won't give away their name here, because they were so kind to me, and infinitely patient. It would be quite wrong of me to make out that their diet didn't work through any fault of their eating plan, or their efforts to make me stick to it.

The diet involved cooking particular recipes for breakfast, lunch and supper. I tried. Oh, how I tried. Mostly low fat and low carbohydrate stuff. It seemed quite sensible to me, nutritionally. But I just cannot stand being told what to eat every day. I seem to rebel against such rigidity.

After two months, Kim, my nanny, had lost a stone and I had put on eight pounds.

Christmas came and went.

And what a peculiar time Christmas is, when you think you're on a diet.

I say 'think' you're on a diet – but actually you're not really, are you? You only kid yourself you are, because you have resolved to yourself so many times that you are 'trying' to lose weight. You start to see Christmas as a real nuisance, which annually threatens to ruin your iron will and perfect self-discipline.

What rubbish I have told myself every Christmas. I start out on December the first, absolutely determined to lose a stone by the 25th, so that I can look wonderful on Christmas day in my little red dress (or whatever!).

By the time I have reached the 15th or so, I haven't lost a pound, because my new diet has been regularly sabotaged by festive parties and seasonal dinners, almost every night.

So I then reckon, if I absolutely starve myself senseless, I can lose ten pounds or so in ten days.

Out of the cupboard comes that battered piece of paper known as my 'emergency soup' recipe, downloaded from the internet a few years ago. It's a sign of how desperate I am by that time of year – the annual ritual of the cabbage soup diet!

Maybe that's why pomanders and cinnamon pot-pourri are so popular at Christmas? It's because every crazy woman in the Christian western world is on a crash diet so that they can look fashionably emaciated on Christmas morning, for drinkies with the relatives.

Funny, though, on Christmas morning, I was exactly the same size as I had been on December the first. No, I lie. I was about two pounds heavier – because after two days of cabbage soup, I lost all reason and ate a freezerful of pizzas. Then, the next day, when I hated myself for giving up, I thought – what the heck, why should I starve myself, I deserve a little TLC: I'll have another pizza, and maybe some garlic bread too.

I don't consistently eat much, you see. Never have. I just have highs and lows. Life recently has been either famine or feast, never a level intake. My body is so confused, it's having a nervous breakdown. No wonder it looks so rough!

January came, and it was time to make some serious New Year resolutions. OK, so I let myself down again this Christmas. But do I really want to look like this, feel like this, *next* Christmas?

I received a belated present from one of my best mates. It was a book called *Slim4Life*, by this guy called Jason Vale.

Can't do me any harm to at least read it, I thought…

I couldn't put it down. I was transfixed. Suddenly I felt I was meeting someone who had a no-nonsense, no gimmick, thoroughly sensible approach to the problems of being overweight. And what's more, the author had been there himself, and won the battle. He had been unhealthy, unfit and overweight, and he was now lithe, lean and energetic. And he had done it without dieting.

I was intrigued.

Having tried every diet ever invented, I was excited by the thought of never trying one again.

But, hang on. The notion of the 'no diet' diet had been around for a while. I had interviewed countless authors (mostly from the States) who recommended ditching the diet books, ending rigid rules about eating and relaxing back and simply 'eating when you are hungry'. Music to my ears!

Of course, I had tried that, too. It resulted in me going wild.

I would order everything on the menu, fill my fridge with cheese, chocolate and delicious French bread, butter and mayonnaise.

Friends would gasp in awe. 'Aren't you on a diet?'

'Yes,' I would smile with understandable satisfaction, as I buttered another cream cracker and tiptoed my way through the cheese board.

'I'm on the no-diet diet! Rigid rules just make me want to break them. This diet says I must relax and eat whatever I want!'

I just lost control! In fact, I had been waiting for this diet all my life!

I first noticed this loss of control over food when I was presenting *Good Morning with Anne and Nick* in the nineties. That was the morning show which was set up by the BBC, quite deliberately to rival Richard and Judy on ITV. My old mate, Nick Owen, and myself were asked to front the two hour show from the Pebble Mill studios in Birmingham, in a studio remodelled from the famous BBC lobby, where they used to present *Pebble Mill at One* and *Saturday Night at the Mill*.

It was a great time. Nick and I had always wanted to work together again since our very happy days at *TV-am*, a decade before. This was like a dream come true – since Nick already lived in Birmingham, and I had always loved the place since I had trained as a TV reporter at ATV/Central.

By 1992, when we went on air from Pebble Mill, my weight was already an issue to me, if no one else. Just in order to shoot the opening sequence, where I was seen walking to the corner shop to buy a bottle of milk, and then popping into the studios where I plonked said bottle of milk down on Nick's desk, I had to diet for three weeks to fit into the suit ordered for me. For the entire sequence, I was sucking my stomach in and trying to smile at the same time.

Only when I found I was pregnant with my fourth child, did I relax about my body. At least I could visibly swell in front of those cameras, without fear of criticism. And so I did – into a large blob with swing pleats and shoulder pads for the majority of the nine-month run.

Jake was born in May 1993, just a few weeks before the entire programme broke for the long summer vacation.

It was crazy, really. The BBC had taken us on to rival *This Morning*, yet every year, just as we had built up a sizeable and loyal following, we were taken off air. Our audience was left high and dry, and free to switch allegiances!

It may have been stupid scheduling, but it was terrific for me, a busy young mother with three small children and a home to run. It meant I could have all summer in the garden with my youngsters. I had the best job in the world!

So, having just given birth, and very tired from a working pregnancy, I unwound for the next few months, and remained in my maternity clothes for weeks and weeks. After all, why rush to get back into shape?

I lounged in the garden, with Jake in the baby bouncer and the other two children, Oliver and Jamie, in the paddling pool beneath a parasol, and I licked the summer away in an overabundance of ice creams.

It was fun, but by the time September came, and morning television was droning with endless coverage of the annual political party conferences, I knew I would soon be returning to work.

I went in for a rummage through my dressing room and the wardrobe lady gasped. Nothing fitted! I stood in front of the mirror with that sinking feeling, hating myself.

What had happened to this once lean, mean presenting machine?

She had got serious motherhood, that's what. She had even bought the T-shirt. Oh yes. And the stretchy leggings. I don't know how those things had suddenly appeared in my wardrobe – but there they were – a pair of black leggings and another pair of navy blue, and even a hideous pair of red ones. Size 14, stretchy. And the T-shirts said 'Large' on the labels.

They cannot be mine, I thought. My Great Aunt Maud must have left a pair of leggings behind when she last visited, and they have bred!

Friends offered their favourite exercise videos for me to borrow. Others suggested diet milk shakes. What about a week away at a health farm?

I did go to one of those posh spas, supposedly for a week.

I drove there, full of hope, dying for a little luxury, pampering and especially looking forward to leaving a stone lighter.

At the beginning of day two, I was utterly miserable. I missed the children so badly – and everyone else there was skinny and gorgeous. I skulked into the steam room, the largest towel available only just covering my blushes, and half a dozen snotty señoritas started chinwagging in Spanish. They were probably gossiping amongst themselves, but I was convinced they were talking about me and my body.

It was the same at the pool. I just felt so huge. I filled my 'treatment card' with appointments all afternoon, and spent my time being pummelled, smothered in seaweed and anointed with emollients.

This will knock me out, I thought, and I'll have a good night's sleep away from demanding kids.

But I spent all night missing them, and hardly grabbed a wink.

So, after my breakfast of muesli and yoghurt, I drove home – an idiotic failure!

My last few days of freedom before another season of *Good Morning with Anne and Nick* were spent panic-dieting. In other words, eating next to nothing and asking people to physically stop me from entering the kitchen.

I just about made it back to a size 12 for the start of the show. But I had a constant struggle with my weight throughout the whole programme run. Every time my waistband felt tight, I would try a different diet.

There was the 'F' plan, the Hay diet, the Scarsdale and those blessed milkshakes, which I ended up drinking with a packet of crisps and a sandwich from the BBC canteen. They were meant to be alternatives to meals – but that only lasted for a few days, after which I treated them as side orders!

Every time I applied myself to a new diet, I would summon all my will power. I was tired and, as winter drew on, I would start shivering in the evenings. That's when I would start to feel a little low – and inevitably I would end up at the fridge door.

(Open my fridge and there would be a little, electronic pig in there, snorting: 'Oh no, you don't! Oh no, you don't!' It was a present from a well-meaning member of the family.)

One night, I picked up the pig and threw it in the waste basket. Its plaintive voice could be heard from inside our wheelie bin by the back door for almost a week, until the bin men came and took it away. It is probably still going, marooned on a land-fill site somewhere in the Midlands, pathetically grunting at scavenging seagulls.

Nothing really seemed to help my battle with the bulge. I couldn't really understand where all this weight was coming from. I did, however, know exactly where it was ending up – mostly on my hips, thighs, and my legs. Well, I hadn't seen my legs for years. They were always inside trousers nowadays. The BBC wardrobe lady desperately tried to tempt me into a skirt – but to no avail.

'I am a trousers person!' I always protested. But deep inside, there was still a girl who longed to be able to wear a bikini and look good in a mini skirt.

Note how I still use the phrase 'be able'? I just said: 'I longed *to be able* to wear a bikini'… 'I longed *to be able* to look good in a mini skirt'… as though some Almighty Power somewhere was stopping me from wearing a bikini. As though it wasn't my own fault; oh no, an outside force, over which I had no control, was preventing me from having the body I really wanted.

That was the first issue that Jason tackled in his book, and the main reason I was hooked until the final page.

He was the first person who looked me in the eyes (if a book can really do that!) and said: 'It's up to you! The buck stops with you. You can do it. It is actually easy, if you know how, if you clear away the fog and open your eyes!'

You just have to re-learn a few basic truths. They are facts which we all know, but many of us have forgotten in this hectic day and age, when we are saturated with media hype and advertising.

In actual fact, those no-diet diets were on the right track. You should bin all those diet books, and get rid of all those stupid rules, regulations and fads which diet inventors claim are the magic key.

You should eat exactly what you want, and eat whenever you are hungry.

What those no-diet dieters didn't add was that, right now, you may not really know or understand precisely what you want and when you are hungry.

This is key. This is crucial.

Don't put this book down now, and go away thinking that all you have got to do is eat what you want when you want. It ain't quite that simple.

You have got to want the right things.

Did you get that?

Let me say it once more, before you go and heat up the oven for that deep-pan pizza, the giant garlic bread and bucket of French fries.

You have got to want the right things. You have got to learn how to love, and desire, and crave the right things, and feel full up, happy and satisfied when you've eaten them.

Then you really can eat when you want, and what you want.

Now if you want the full details, and all the knowledge, then you must read Jason's book, or get yourself along to one of his seminars (details at www.thejuicemaster.com) where he spells it all out in glorious, technicolour demonstrations. He is a guy with the gift of the gab – you know? He talks like an American, with evangelistic enthusiasm and his message is contagious – easy to catch! You'll find it fascinating.

But let me run through it all briefly here for you to taste. Here's the basic idea:

You see, really good food is good for you, and eating nothing but good food will put you back on track, make you healthy, and lose you weight – because it is what nature intended you to eat.

Eating when you are hungry is the natural way. It is the only reason you should eat.

BUT:

We have been so brainwashed by the advertising and hype of the modern food industry, that we have come, over a lifetime's indoctrination, to regard a load of ill-nourishing, processed rubbish as desirable.

We buy orange-coloured sugary liquid for ourselves and our kids, in the misguided belief that it has come from an orange. The advertising cleverly suggests it is real orange juice, but in fact, it never says so. You'd have to read the label. Chances are, it may never have seen an orange grove in its life – which in fact started in a laboratory. But it is packed with sugar, so your children will love it (we are all born with an innate liking for sweet taste) and they'll ask you to buy more.

We think bread is the 'staff of life' and yet most of us buy a loaf of plasticated slices made from flour which has had all the good stuff (the wholegrains with all the vitamins and minerals) taken out, in order to prolong its shelf life. Profit matters more than nutrition, you see. Once you know that fact, you are staggered that it's allowed.

We think roast chicken crisps have been flavoured with roast chicken. But look on the back of the packet. 'Suitable for vegetarians', it says. Huh? How come? Because they can synthesise the taste, with chemicals!

To suit our busy lifestyles, we buy ready meals which boast a long list of chemical additives. We even buy meat products which have had all the flavour factory-farmed out of them, and then sugar added to put a tempting flavour back in.

Heck, according to a recent *Panorama,* you can even buy a chicken breast nowadays which has been so mangled by man that it contains an additive (which causes it to absorb water, and so weigh more) that is made from pork. Thus your innocent and healthy-looking chicken actually contains pig DNA.

The truth is that eating large quantities of fatty, processed, refined, sweetened foodstuff is not healthy for you. For that reason, it can make you put on weight because you can easily overeat calorie dense foods without realising it.

Some people seem to be able to keep things in perspective. Others of us become victims of a food madness without realising it, and without knowing how to rescue ourselves.

I thought that I shopped, cooked and ate healthily. But I was also hooked on to the bad stuff that makes you eat too much, too often, without even realising.

I am a vegetarian (well, not strictly – I do eat fish. But I will use the term here for convenience). I thought that, because I ate a lot of home-cooked meals, I must be eating the best.

But when I really analysed my food eating, and I wrote it all down, I found I was wrong.

I was hooked particularly on refined carbohydrates – white pasta, white rice, white bread, biscuits, crackers, rice cakes, crisps.

At around eight every evening I would begin to crave carbs, and I would cook myself a mountain of white rice or white pasta, complete with a vegetable stir-fry topped off with a tin of creamy mushroom sauce.

Sometimes I didn't even bother with the sauce. I would just have a pile of pasta with a little grated cheese on the top.

What's wrong with that? Perfectly healthy!

But refined pasta and rice have been processed, stripped from their wholegrain jackets, so that some important vitamins and minerals and fibre are thrown away as if they were worthless individuals. More importantly, removing fibre means that the carbohydrates from refined foods are broken down easily and rapidly causing a rush of sugar into the bloodstream. Since our bodies are delicate machines which don't like extreme highs or lows of sugar, insulin is produced; this hormone acts to bring the sugar levels down to normal. Unfortunately in order to do this, any excess sugar is taken up by our body cells and ultimately converted and stored as fat.

I was doing the very worst thing with the very best of intentions – because I simply didn't know enough about the food I was eating, and what it was doing to me.

Suddenly, things started to make sense.

Knowledge is power.

Knowledge empowers you to make the right decisions for yourself, your body.

Knowing what's in a food, and what it might do for you, or to you, will inevitably help you make the right decisions.

Knowledge, real knowledge, will turn you right off the bad stuff. Remember my sausage story. Once I knew what was in them, I never wanted another.

It reminds me of a trip Nick Owen and I took to Los Angeles, to present a programme about the 25th anniversary of Mickey Mouse!

It was the first time either of us had ever flown first-class.

After we had stopped celebrity spotting in the exclusive cabin, we settled down to supper. No food trays and plastic cutlery here. This was all silver service. While we sipped champagne, and tried to look as though we flew in style all the time, we chose from the menu.

Our camera crew was travelling with us. The cameraman filmed while we ordered.

Starters were either caviar or pâté de foie gras.

I chose pâté – those were the days before I had become veggie. I knew I liked the taste, but I didn't really know anything about foie gras.

That was until, weeks later, the letters of complaint and protest came flooding into my office at *TV-am*.

Viewers were outraged. Didn't I know how pâté de foie gras was made? Many letters included leaflets with appalling pictures of geese being force fed, their beaks wired open and funnels shoved down their throats, literally stuffed with food so that their livers would almost explode – so producing the upmarket delicacy.

Once I had seen those pictures, and read the truth, I could barely believe such a practice was allowed in this day and age. I had had no idea. The cruelty defies imagination. How anyone could eat the stuff, knowing where it came from, bewilders me.

I have never, ever touched pâté de foie gras again. Like those sausages, I have lived without foie gras quite happily – I have not missed eating it, I have not craved it, I do not feel deprived without it.

So knowledge can turn your appetite right off. It can dramatically change your choices.

If a little knowledge can make me do a U turn on sausages and pâté de foie gras – what could it do for my whole eating lifestyle?

I changed my mind again. This time I decided that, yes, I would love to meet Jason, the Juice Master!

We met in my mate's kitchen. Jason was juicing. To his right, he had an enormous pile of pineapples, apples, avocados, carrots, cucumbers, peppers, celery and other assorted fruits and veggies. On his left, he was feeding stuff into the juicer, which was roaring away at full speed.

Minutes later, he poured a vibrant yellow liquid into tall glasses, and toasted our health.

It was the beginning of the end for me. The end of the diet disasters. The light at the end of the tunnel.

The opening of a new chapter in my life.

Ten reasons why diets don't work

Every time I have embarked on a 'diet', I have lost a little weight for the first few days. *Then*, I have despaired. *Then* I have given up. *Then* I have put on more weight. It's the classic yo-yo syndrome. Here are ten good reasons why diets don't work.

1. Diets don't address the problem

Why are you overweight? Probably because, over many years, you have developed inappropriate eating habits. Obesity is a problem caused by our modern eating habits in the Western world. Diets answer this problem by telling us to eat in an even crazier manner – cutting things out, denying ourselves foods we crave – and then finally abandoning us to the habits which caused the problem in the first place.

2. Diets teach us nothing but food phobia

We all know that when you are on diet, all you can think of is food. You become obsessed about what you are 'allowed' to eat. Diets teach us to portion control,

weigh and analyse our food and constantly juggle calorie values in our heads –
without taking into account the nutritional value. That's why some diets would
rather you ate an ice cream than a yoghurt – yet the latter is often lower in fat
and calories. Some experts now think an obsession with dieting can lead to
eating disorders.

3. Diets are so negative

Diets are so awful because they are like a punishment – not a solution. You feel
constantly deprived and depressed. How many times have you moaned out loud
in a café or restaurant: 'I can't have that, because I am on a diet.' Diets are all
about what you cannot have, what you cannot do. No wonder so many people
give up – that's no way to live!

4. Diets are unrealistic, unnatural and unpleasant

That's why 95% of dieters fail. For a start, they advertise themselves using
Hollywood actresses who have never had a weight problem in their lives! Then
they tell you that you can lose up to two pounds a day – or some such claim. But
how many people can realistically do that? Then, once the hope has got you
hooked, they tell you to give up eating all the things you love. Telling you to live on
calorie-counted processed gunk or milk shakes, or only combining certain foods
with certain others, artificially cutting out carbs or fat or all dairy products, is just
unreal – and we live in the real world.

5. Diets cause loss in muscle as well as fat

Low-calorie diets cause you to lose both muscle and fat. However, when you
eventually gain back the weight, (and remember 95% of us do), it is all fat and not
muscle, causing your metabolism to slow down even more. Now you have extra
weight, but less muscle.

6. Diets are physically and emotionally stressful

As if life weren't hard enough! A huge part of the dieting problem is
depression. If you have tried diet after diet, and you are still fat, then you are
bound to feel depressed. What's more, you probably take emotional refuge in

food – so just when you feel you need propping up by munching on a tube of choc chip cookies, you find they're banned. And then you feel even more desperate, and stressed. What is more likely to drive you towards the biscuit cupboard?

7. Diets make you put your life on hold

In my job, I have been so lucky to be invited out to wonderful social events. But I have turned down so many in the past few years because I have thought I will wait until I am a size 12. It happened for Liz Taylor's fiftieth birthday party. I turned it down because I knew I would have to look good and I felt fat. By the time Liz Taylor was sixty, I was a size 12 and she wasn't in Britain for her birthday. Learn from my lesson. Dieters are life-long procrastinators. Give it all up now, today, and start living tonight!

8. Diets make you miserable company

Pity the family and friends of the yo-yo dieter. They go to the fridge for a snack – and find it stuffed with 'lite', 'low cal' margarines, yoghurts and ready meals, and they quite rightly moan that it's tasteless rubbish. You moan all the time about what you cannot have, and your friends are fed up hearing it. You cast a depressive low on every social event you do agree to go to. You give waiters a hard time about what ingredients they must leave out of the dish, you make it awkward for dinner party hostesses to know what to give you. Don't make yourself a diet bore.

9. Diets make you weak

Just when you need to be exercising more, and getting fit! Most diets have one thing in common, even though they might dress it up some other way – they are usually very low in calories. This may, if you can stick to it, lose you pounds, but it will also make you feel very weak. (And cold – I always get so cold in the evenings when I am on a diet. Then I end up spoiling the diet regime by eating something purely to warm me up.) Yet this is a time when you also need to get fit – because exercise fuels your metabolism and muscles burn calories just by existing.

10. Diets make you fat

When you go on a low-calorie diet, your body thinks you are starving; it actually becomes more efficient at storing fat by slowing down your metabolism. When you stop this unrealistic eating plan, your metabolism is still slow and inefficient – so that you gain the weight back even faster, even though you may still be eating less than you were before you went on the diet.

chapter 3

emotional eating

I wasn't overweight, though, just because of refined, processed and convenience foods. In fact, in the past few years I had been doing lots of home cooking. Yes, I was undoubtedly a refined carbohydrate addict. I just loved pizzas, pastas, bread and absolutely anything to do with rice.

I was a midnight muncher and a comfort eater – and I think that was probably my biggest problem. One of my favourite quick and easy meals was a mountain of fresh white spaghetti, covered with a creamy onion and mushroom sauce, made with just a little butter, herbs and crème fraîche.

That sounds like a great dinner, I hear you say.

Maybe, but not at one o'clock in the morning. And that is quite often the time I would start cooking. When all the children had gone to bed, and the house was quiet, and my thoughts were at last my own, I would hover in the kitchen, doing all of those little tidying-up chores you do before putting the house to sleep, and then quite suddenly I would find myself chopping onions and mushrooms, ready for the frying pan.

Sometimes in the school holidays, my children and I would love to stay up very late at night, and have a midnight feast. I must have been teaching them appalling habits for later life. Thankfully, I think they have inherited their father's genes rather than mine when it comes to physique – so they'll probably never have a weight problem. But midnight feasts are such fun, aren't they? Fine, as long as you don't make it a habit!

I had always been fairly adamant that I ate healthy food. I was a vegetarian, except that I did, and still do, eat fish. I loved the basic carbohydrates – white bread, white pasta and white rice dishes. I had long given up using butter apart from the small amount that goes into my midnight spaghetti snack. I didn't take sugar in my coffee or on breakfast cereals. And, unlike many of my friends, I wasn't addicted to sweet desserts and chocolate. (Although, if offered, I always said yes to second helpings – of anything! I think that relates back to being told as a child that I must eat everything on my plate, and think of the starving children in the Congo.)

Only when I carefully wrote down a food diary, did I start to see a pattern emerge that might help to explain just why I had put on weight.

I lived in the kitchen.

Any mum does, I suppose, particularly if you have a lot of children, and they always seem to be hungry. During school holidays, it seems that there is hardly a five minute gap between washing up after one meal and chopping, mashing and catering the next.

Only mothers in glossy magazines get up, get dressed, and go downstairs to read, or assemble a jigsaw with little Freddie, for an hour or so in the living room or conservatory. The rest of us fall out of bed, slide downstairs and only wake up propped up over a strong coffee in the kitchen. That's certainly how it was for me!

Minutes after I'd descended, the hordes would come down for their various forms of breakfast. I would have a slice or two of toast, with one son, a bowl of cereal with another, then some fruit (to encourage another), all punctuated with even stronger cups of coffee.

I used to look forward to elevenses. Coffee and biscuits – no matter where I was, working or not. Elevenses took me back to a time when I was training to be a TV reporter at the BBC, in London. That was back in the days when the BBC still employed trolley ladies. You would be sitting at your typewriter, bashing away at a news story, and then you would hear the tinkle, rattle, thump and shoosh of the incoming tea lady. And she always had Kit Kats – lots of them.

A cup of BBC tea and a large Kit Kat were one of the highlights of the day. Apart from midnight feasts, I think 'elevenses' is the best meal of the day. Why did I so much look forward to those, when I cannot even remember a really great lunch or tea time?

I'd probably still be in therapy this time next year if I really wanted to find out why. But you can see a pattern building, can't you? I loved eating certain foods, at certain times of day, in order to give me a particular mood.

I was a mood foodie.

I ate, not because I was hungry, but because I was after an emotional response.

I was an emotional eater.

What's the bet that you are, too?

Because, if you really look at it, hardly any of us in the affluent West ever get hungry. We eat because society has told us to eat three times a day and we eat for social purposes. We meet friends for a coffee and a cake – we don't meet for a gossip on the street corner. When we meet a new suitor, they take us out for dinner. We invite friends around for drinks and snacks. We use eating as a passport to socialising.

We are *always* eating!

Then there are the times when we eat for comfort. I know I did. Any little problem, and I would retire to the biscuit cupboard. I could get through an entire day of 'being good' diet-wise, and then as soon as all the chores were done, the meals finished, tidied and washed up, the kids put to bed, I would get out the comfort food.

I think it was a big mistake putting a TV in the kitchen. Or having a kitchen that was a little too comfortable – so you would never be more than an arm's length from teatime leftovers! Food must be one of the most instantly comforting things there is in life. I suppose because it is the ultimate nurturing, life-sustaining substance. More important even than love.

Now there's a deep statement – but one which is bandied about such a lot, if only in joke. Just how many surveys have there been, which have asked women the question: 'Is food/chocolate more important than sex?' And the overwhelming answer has always been – yes!

It's because so many women have an emotional relationship with food. We don't just see it as sustenance. It is not something which is just ingested when we are hungry. For a start, it's the ultimate gift we can give to our children (other than life itself). We are programmed to worry about feeding our young. We feel thrilled to see our culinary offerings polished off by our family. We feel utterly rejected and upset if the little ratbags turn up their noses at our efforts.

Toddlers know they can twist us around their little fingers by being awkward over food – because it matters so much to us! A man will witness the tantrums and remark: 'Don't worry about it. Little Freddie will eat when he is hungry enough!' But we women wither and die at the very thought he has missed a meal.

Food is that important to us. It goes to the very core of our emotional well-being, our ability to be a good mother, a good wife, a superwoman. Added on to all that is the brainwashing we have endured since childhood. How often were we told: 'Be a good girl, and you can have some sweets!'

Food is often used in our society as a reward for good behaviour – and often the worst, sugary food, too!

I cannot tell you why some women have always managed to keep these things in perspective, and others haven't. And until now, I would have always denied that I was an emotional eater. But I do accept now that I am – or at least, I was.

Emotional eaters will swear that certain foods, or eating at certain times, makes them feel better.

But I had to ask myself this question: Does it really?

Did I feel happier once I had downed a mountain of mushroom pasta in the middle of the night?

Did I feel more able to cope after my eleven o'clock tea and Kit Kat?

Did it make me feel more contented to spend the evening curled up in the kitchen, nibbling whatever came to hand?

At first, I found myself answering – 'well, actually – yes!'

But the truth is that the satisfaction from the food was very, very short-lived. Yes, I suppose the injection of sugar from the Kit Kat (and all the other foods) would have quickly given me a sugar 'high' which might have meant a short burst of energy. But, a quick sugar fix is followed by a low, usually resulting in wanting more food more quickly.

And there's no doubt that, shortly after eating those comfort foods, I wanted to kick myself up the backside for eating them. So they really weren't a comfort at all. In fact, they simply added to my problem. I just fancied them because I thought they would be comforting.

It's not all our fault, either.

So many foods (particularly chocolate bars and fast foods like burgers) are especially marketed with 'instant gratification' messages. Not only do they promise you instant relief from hunger, they also suggest that, by eating the foodstuff, you'll reach a new level of consciousness, one where you float high above the clouds, where you'll meet your dream man (sex is used to sell a lot of chocolate – have you noticed?).

I'm not suggesting for a minute that we are all so stupid that we actually believe this is all going to happen just because we bite into a flaky chocolate bar. But it's all about perception, isn't it? Chocolate means luxury. Luxury means treating ourselves, because we deserve it. So we say – why not? I deserve a little pampering!

And so we allow ourselves a food which the advertising industry tells us is a luxury. Whereas in fact, it's loaded with saturated fat and refined sugar, designed to pile on the pounds and make us want to eat more. And then regret it afterwards!

The other emotional reason many people blame for eating is boredom. Yet eating doesn't solve boredom – it merely fills the time, as it fills your stomach. Boredom has nothing to do with food. If you really are bored, then you need to find something to do – and there are a million things you could probably do which would keep you so busy you wouldn't have time to eat.

Depression is another big reason for eating – yet again, food doesn't help, in fact, it ultimately makes things worse. If you are upset or low – look for the real reason and try to address that. You are not depressed because your food stocks are low, therefore it makes no sense to stock them up!

So to put it bluntly: eating for emotional comfort rather than to satisfy hunger, or turning to food when you're stressed, upset, anxious or excited means that you lose control over what you eat and therefore eat far more than you would physiologically need. This results in a cycle of gaining weight and then getting depressed, which leads to more eating, thus creating a self-perpetuating cycle.

Bad habits are yet another reason for overeating.

I can come in from a long day at work, my feet are killing me, I am hot, sweaty and tired, and my eyes are strained, my voice hoarse and I feel all sorts of aches and pains after being slumped in the car for a two hour drive home.

And what do I do?

I make straight for the kitchen. Well, it is like Bush Telegraph Central in our house. It's where you go to find out the latest gossip – who's done what at school, who is still doing homework, who has telephoned today etc. But, as subconsciously as breathing, my fingers do the walking – to the fridge. And suddenly, I am nibbling something I shouldn't. Half a bit of leftover pizza, a couple of cold veggie bangers, and cheese and biscuits. Very often they don't even taste very nice. But walking in, feeling 'I'm home at last!' and nibbling something is a vital ritual.

In fact, once I started writing these things down, I noticed that I eat something every single time I enter the kitchen. And since I do that several hundred times a day, it's not surprising to find that it all adds up!

Other mums I have spoken to say they simply have to eat when their children do. Again, it is a ritual, a habit.

If you have bad food habits – then that is all they are, mere habits. They can be easily changed, or replaced by better habits. In fact, that's the key.

So how do you change your eating patterns if you are an emotional eater? It is simpler than you think. I know, because I have made the change – and it doesn't mean you are an emotional nutcase and you have got to solve all your little emotional problems overnight.

In fact, you haven't got to address the emotions at all.

All you have got to do is understand, and believe, that food will not solve those problems.

So stop trying to address those emotions with food. Address them with something else. Change your habits by replacing them with new, different ones. It's incredibly logical – and it is not as hard to do as it may seem.

Look at me.

I was a midnight muncher. Now, having read lots of research on the subject, I understand that I was midnight feasting for several reasons.

1. I had made it a habit, and my sleeping pattern had adapted to it.
2. I thought, wrongly (because I quickly regretted it), that it would make me feel good.
3. I thought I was hungry.
4. I thought the food I was eating was healthy.
5. I thought it was fun.

Right – let's see the truth:

1. Yes, it was a habit – but it wasn't doing my sleep any good. I often slept heavier after a big meal, and woke up lethargic.
2. I regretted eating the food almost as soon as I had eaten the last mouthful.
3. I wasn't hungry. I just 'fancied' it!
4. I was actually eating a big pile of refined, white pasta. That stuff, as we have already learned, is a refined carb – it causes blood sugar to spike, insulin to rush in and excess calories to be deposited in the body as fat. And, at that time of night, every calorie is excess, since your body only needs enough energy to see it through the night. I was eating enough to sustain a marathon runner in a big race.
5. Given the above, it's a strange sort of fun, isn't it? I wanted to lose weight. I hated being fat – and yet I thought eating too much in the middle of the night was *fun*?

In fact, the midnight munchies is now a well-documented eating disorder. One recent study in the USA reckons that we midnight munchers do so because we feel less inhibited by dim lighting and the quiet solace of late night. They have found that keeping the lights on full blast in the houses of midnight munchers significantly reduces the amount of times they venture downstairs to eat!

I certainly had an emotional relationship with food. I would turn to safe, cosy sorts of foods if ever anything went wrong in my life. I used to call it nursery food – you know? The types of food you only find in homes with small kids. And, naturally, you associated them with your own childhood, so they conjured up feelings of hearth and home, security and safety.

Things like mince and mashed potato. Toad in the Hole. Fish fingers and chips. Jam sarnies. Neapolitan ice cream with tinned peaches! Choc ices! The list goes on. I am sure you can add to it very easily!

Well, without wishing to go into too many gory details, I did have a decade of almighty highs and thoroughly dreadful lows. In just a few years, I lost my son, my father and then my husband. Food was a great comfort at certain dark times of the night, I can tell you. I don't seek to proffer it as an excuse – it's just a fact. But spending the nineties on an emotional roller coaster means I am very determined to cruise through the early years of the new millennium on a straight and even path.

And my appalling food habits? Well, you don't need to be a psycho-therapist nor a dietician to realise that if I had come in from a hard day at work, I would have been far better off had I gone straight upstairs for a long soak in the bath – and not for a binge in the kitchen.

I simply had to identify those bad habits, and choose other things to do instead.

And if I can do it, anyone can.

Quiz. Do you try to eat your problems away?

1. You have had a terrible day. The boss at work yelled at you. The train home was late. It rained until your hair was flat, your new jacket soaked through and your shoes leaked. At home, the whole family is bad tempered and no one seems to care about your woes. Do you:

A: Empty the freezer and cook an enormous fry-up of eggs, bacon, sausages, beans and fried potatoes!

B: Pour yourself a drink, grab a snack and unwind in front of the TV.

C: Go straight upstairs for a long, hot bath and enjoy some relaxing music.

2. You are sitting up in bed, watching the late night movie *Gone With The Wind*. Blue has just died, Rhett Butler has walked out, Scarlett O'Hara is bereft and you suddenly feel the need for chocolate – but there is none. Do you:

A: Get dressed, climb into the car and drive to your nearest all-night garage to buy some?

B: Turn the house upside down looking for chocolate in all your secret hiding places?

C: Promise yourself you'll have some tomorrow, and watch the end of the movie.

3. You're trying to diet – and you agree that, if you stick to the rules for just one day, you will treat yourself. Would that treat be:

A: A chocolate bar.

B: A piece of fruit.

C: An aromatherapy bath with a face-pack.

4. When you were a little girl, how did your mother reward good behaviour?

A: She said you could have sweets.

B: She gave you extra pocket money.

C: She told you how much she appreciated you.

5. You have been dieting like mad, and you have just lost your first stone. Congratulations! How are you going to celebrate?

A: We are going out for a slap-up celebration meal.

B: I am going to buy a new piece of clothing – one I couldn't fit into before.

C: I am going to take my best friend for a day at our local health spa.

6. You have won a competition and the prize is a weekend at a luxury hotel. As soon as you check in, you're invited to the restaurant for dinner on the house. You have already eaten at home, and you are not hungry. Do you:

A: Eagerly accept and order a lavish meal – after all, it is even more tasty when it is free!

B: Politely decline, but ask for a drink and canapés in your room instead.

C: Eagerly accept, and just nibble at a light salad.

7. You have been doing really well on your diet and then today, you found yourself at lunch eating fish and chips, followed by an enormous chocolate fudge sundae. After so many days of discipline, you have just blown it. Do you:

A: Eat a Chinese takeaway for tea, a box of chocolates for supper and fry up a midnight feast, thinking, 'I've blown this diet, so I'll just have to try another on Monday.'

B: Spend the rest of the day in misery, hopping on the scales and worrying.

C: Get back on track straight away by having a light salad or a smoothie for supper.

8. You have just been asked out to dinner by a gorgeous man. He's taking you to one of the best eateries in town. Do you:

A: Eat next to nothing – you want to show him you're a dainty little thing.

B: Order your favourite meal – you want to relax and really enjoy yourself.

C: Not even think about food.

9. You have just had a blazing row with your partner. Do you:

A: Slam the door on him and bury yourself in the biscuit cupboard.

B: Cook him his favourite meal as a way of saying sorry.

C: Wait for a while, then try to talk it through with him.

10. You were going out bowling tonight, but it's been called off. All your friends are off doing other things, your mum isn't answering the phone, there's nothing good on the TV, and the book you've been reading is a little dull. You're bored. Do you:

A: Get out a recipe book and cook yourself an exciting dinner for one.

B: Go to bed early.

C: Go to the gym – there's always someone interesting there!

How did you do?

Mostly As

You are a diet victim. It probably started when you were little – with the wrong sort of reinforcement, like your parents giving you sweets for good behaviour. We don't know we're doing it at the time, but we are teaching kids to associate sugary treats with luxury, as a positive force, when in fact they're bad for us! That's why, now you're an adult, you are more likely to comfort eat and inevitably wreck every diet you ever start. Food is a constant problem for you: one minute it's a luxury, the next it's a nightmare. At times, you even act like a junkie in need of a fix. (I remember raiding my kids' Easter eggs one night, and then denying everything the next morning!) You associate your love life with food – you see a box of chocolates as a sign of love, and then hate yourself for eating them. You even think about the way you eat your food as a romantic 'turn on' or 'turn off' when you're taken out to dinner. But food shouldn't be an emotional tool – it's just food. If you are feeling unhappy, miserable, lonely or bored – that is nothing to do with food. You cannot eat problems away. In fact, eating often makes them worse. Instead, find out what's making you bored, lonely or upset, and address that. You've got to try to separate your eating habits from your emotional ones, or food will always be your master and you its slave. And are slaves ever happy?

Mostly Bs

You have an emotional relationship with food. It is not ruling your life – yet. However, you need to learn to separate the two things – how you feel emotionally should have nothing to do with how you eat, except on the hopefully rare occasions when we simply cannot eat because we are very upset or frightened. You curl up in front of the TV with a drink and nibbles to cheer yourself up after a hard day, when in fact you'd be far better off taking a long hot bath and changing your mood. Don't address your mood with food!

You are also still hooked on the idea of having 'good' and 'bad' days on a diet. You are obsessed with the scales, and see a piece of fruit as a treat for a 'good' diet day. Of course, fruit is lovely, nutritious, and a far better option than chocolate. But you have got to stop seeing food of any sort as a reward. You are losing weight quite well, but you still try to reward 'good' dieting with shopping therapy! You would be far better off going along to a health spa with a friend – because that is a positive way of looking forward to a new, healthier life. And don't shut yourself in your bedroom with a private drink and canapés – do the same social things that everyone else does, just learn how to do them without eating emotionally!

Mostly Cs

The only person I know who is as brilliant as you is Jason Vale – and he has been learning how to eat and exercise healthily for years!

Seriously, if you have answered mostly Cs, then you are definitely on the right track to a New You. You have learned how to separate food from your emotions, and you have made a new habit of answering your moods by changing your behaviour – like going out, doing some exercise or addressing what is really wrong instead of trying to solve a problem with food. People who are truly slim and fit don't spend much time thinking about food at all – that's the true freedom – and you're nearly there!

How to stop comfort eating

So you're a comfort eater – take some real comfort from changing your ways!

Well, congratulations on at least one positive point – if you're an emotional eater, it means you are a highly sensitive person who is in tune with her feelings. (Or at least, that's what I keep telling myself. Better than being a cold-hearted fish, ain't it?)

Comfort eating is when you eat simply to fill up the huge void within yourself. You feel emptiness inside, and try to fill it with food. The trouble is, you are eating with your emotions, responding to your highs and lows with food as a sort of therapy.

Traditionally, foods like chocolate and ice cream are 'comfort foods', but sometimes anything will do. You know you are not hungry, but you eat anyway. Whether angry, upset, needing a retreat from the big bad world, or just plain bored, breaking the diet and stuffing your face is a common form of release.

If food has been your anaesthetic, then to cure emotional overeating you will need to bear some discomfort – the discomfort of saying what you are *really* feeling, the discomfort of an argument, or the discomfort of someone clashing with you. Learning how to stop overeating and putting this into practice will energise you, improve digestion, help you sleep better, boost self-confidence and allow you to be healthier. And you'll feel empowered. Acknowledging these benefits and realising that you want them to be a part of your life will enable you to be happier eating less.

It often comes down to stress. Food is your edible tranquilliser. In fact, that's true. Foods that are rich in carbohydrates increase levels of serotonin in the brain, and serotonin minimises symptoms of stress. That's why you feel that a quick packet of biscuits will make you feel better. In fact it will, but not in the long run if you are trying to lose weight! And if you are trying to slim with one of those very low-carbohydrate diets like The Zone or the Atkins, you will have an even harder time sticking to it if you are under stress. Because these diets that are low in carbohydrates cause a reduction of brain serotonin, and low serotonin levels are themselves associated with insomnia, tension and anxiety.

So now you have got to do for yourself what any therapist would do: you've got to analyse when you eat, in what circumstances, and decide what are the triggers for your eating. Only then can you deduce why you comfort eat, and only after that can you figure out a way to change your habits.

Step 1:

Write down everything you eat in a notebook and include everything, even snacks and drinks. (This is what brought me face to face with what I was really doing.) Also make a note of the time you eat, what you eat, the quantity, feelings of hunger and your mood (are you bored, stressed, nervous, frustrated, angry, sad, happy or lonely?). You have no idea how much you can learn simply by keeping a food diary for a week. But be honest with yourself or it's a waste of time!

Step 2:

Analyse your week. Look at the food you ate when you weren't actually hungry or it wasn't a mealtime. Were you upset over something? Depressed? Or perhaps just low through exhaustion, worry or boredom. What were you doing when you succumbed to that packet of biscuits? Which room were you in? The kitchen? Or maybe, like lots of women, you've found that sitting in front of the TV is the regular trigger for eating.

Step 3:

Now think about what things make you feel better, cheer you up almost immediately – that are not food. Maybe you love taking a long, hot bath? Or playing some music? Reading a book, popping around to a friend's house? Watching a favourite videotape movie? And don't say, having a quick drink, because alcohol is an appetite stimulant and a mood depressant, so having a quick glass of wine will actually make things worse. Think of five or six ideas for upping your mood.

Step 4:

Now put those ideas into practice. Each time you find yourself about to stuff something into your mouth, ask yourself if you are really hungry. If you say yes, eat and enjoy what you want to eat. Savour every mouthful – don't just stuff it in. If on the other hand your body says no, stop and think of your list of ideas – go and have an aromatherapy bath, quick! Perhaps you could take that walk or ring a friend, or better still do twenty minutes exercise – that will automatically make you feel better, because it releases endorphins, the body's feelgood chemical. Continue with the food diary so that you can see how your habits gradually improve.

Remember that situations, not hunger, trigger a comfort eater's desire to overeat – particularly their favourite comfort foods. But you don't have to give up foods that make you feel better, you just need to break the pattern of out-of-control eating, or eating for the wrong reasons at the wrong time.

If you know that you are prone to eat more when you are stressed, here are some tips that experts recommend to help you keep control:

- Don't eat comfort foods that are high in fat – or only eat them in moderate amounts.
- Don't skip meals: you are more likely to overeat at dinner if you pass on breakfast and lunch.
- Pay attention to eating a balanced diet.
- Eliminate eating in front of the TV.
- Look for ways to include physical activity in your daily life.
- Find ways other than eating to relieve stress and anxiety.
- Try to be aware of what your personal overeating triggers are.

The most important thing to know is – comfort eating isn't a food problem, it's an emotional one. If you can find what it is that triggers the behaviour in you, try to solve the underlying problem. If you're bored, find something to do; if depressed, find something to cheer yourself up or seek help from your GP. If you think it's a case of plain bad habits, take up a new hobby: take up painting (as I did!), or enrol for an evening course, or paint the ceiling or take up knitting. If you don't have a DIY job to do, you are a rare breed indeed. Come to my house – I could keep you busy for a year!

chapter 4

eating healthily – for life

OK – so you now want to know what the rules and regulations of this diet actually are. What foods you are allowed and what is banned. When and how often you are allowed to have meals.

The truth is – there are no rules, nothing is banned. You eat what you want to eat. You eat when you are hungry. You don't have to count calories, combine food types, add up points or weigh fat grams.

Sounds too good to be true? Well, of course there is a catch.

The catch is – it will only work for you, slim you down, make you feel healthier, fitter and more lively, *if you understand and believe what we've already learned about food.*

If you still want to eat refined and processed foods, those with all the goodness taken out, too much salt and refined sugar added in; if you still want to drink carbonated liquid sugars which later make you feel thirstier; if you still want to eat to try to comfort some deep-rooted unhappiness, or eat too much out of habit; if you still do the midnight munchies even though it depresses you – then you might as well not read the next bit!

Because the buck stops here.

I was at a meeting a couple of years ago, organised by the women's magazine *Woman's Own*. They had assembled a group of readers who all desperately wanted to lose weight. Over a period of 12 weeks, the magazine would follow their trials and tribulations, and see if their willpower, combined with some expert guidance, would help them lose weight.

At the first get-together, we met nutritionist Amanda Ursell.

The first message she wanted to get across to the magazine's 'Dream Bodies' (for so they were called!) was that the only person who could make the difference was… yourself. No one else!

Yes, of course, experts could inform and guide. But they could only arm you with the truth about food and why some of us are overweight. They couldn't diet for you.

All good weight loss counsellors talk about it nowadays. They call it 'taking responsibility' for your weight.

You see, so many people embark upon a diet with the very best of intentions. They willingly submit themselves to a rigid, and sometimes highly complicated, list of rules and restrictions. They meekly accept that they will only be able to eat certain foods at certain times of the day. They give up control of their eating to whoever invented the latest diet fad.

So when everything goes pear-shaped, and it all ends in disaster – the dieter doesn't have to think of blaming herself – she can just blame the man in the white coat who thought up the whole hare-brained scheme!

Many overeaters, especially those who have spent years dieting, like to think about food in terms of what they are or aren't allowed to eat. This prohibitive thinking creates rules and restrictions that make them think negatively about eating. They think, 'I mustn't eat any more biscuits, so I'll be good and put the packet away.' That's being 'good'. Or: 'I know I shouldn't eat any more, but I'm going to be naughty and have another biscuit.' That's being a rebel!

I have to confess, that was me! I just saw a diet as a load of rules I could make a point of breaking.

Being compliant may work in the short-term and is usually how diets work when they are successful. But compliance often encourages rebellion later and most people who rebel end up not only going off their diet altogether, but often feel as if their eating is more out of control than before they started dieting. Compliance to the 'rules' – even if you stick to them and lose some weight – doesn't work in the long term anyway, because you don't learn how to eat for the rest of your life. Once you decide to give up the rules, you go back to your old ways.

What you have got to do is accept – from this moment onwards – that you must take responsibility for whatever you eat from now on. That means that you will decide whether or not you are going to eat.

The choice is yours. Instead of complying with the rules and regulations of a diet, acknowledge that you are completely free to eat anything and everything you want. Making yourself – not a diet – responsible for what you eat will help you make the best decisions about food. Because you are in control of your choices, you won't feel deprived, you will actually feel free.

Free to eat healthily. You know what the healthy foods are now. Eat as many as you *really want*. Eat for the only good reason we should eat – *because we are hungry*. Do that, and you will eat healthily, you will lose weight and feel better and fitter.

Hey – just let me say that again:

You are free!

Free to eat whatever you really, really want. I just hope that, like me, you are beginning to change your mind about what you really, really do want.

Remember the sausages and the pâté de foie gras? How I was utterly put off them once I knew the facts about them.

Well, I am free to eat as many sausages and as much pâté de foie gras as I want.

I just don't want them any more. I can say 'no, thanks', because they mean nothing to me. Well, OK, sausages still smell good when I first catch a whiff of them sizzling in the pan. But within a split second my brain is telling me what it is that's causing that aroma (saturated fat and frying offal) – and I can happily ignore what others find tempting.

It's great!

Now, I know it sounds a bit like adopting a new religion. Believe, and you will find the way forward! Give up the wicked ways of the past, and you will be saved!

I think that's because the message is so simple, that it sounds almost daft to say it aloud.

We human beings are meant to eat as Mother Nature intended. Eat healthily and you'll be healthy. You are what you eat. Go back to basics.

But, hey, we all live in a modern world – and if you are anything like me, you need it all spelled out a bit more clearly than that.

So here goes.

The facts to remember are:

1. Diets don't work. They just make you obsessed about food. They fail 95% of the time. They turn you into a lifelong moaner and yo-yo dieter!

2. It feels great to be fit. You have to start slowly and build – doing any activity that suits you. You don't have to be a fanatic, just a little movement every day – and even I got to like it!

3. Much of our food is spoiled by processing or refining. Many nutrients are removed in order to improve the products' shelf life

and appearance – eating large quantities of refined and processed foods can encourage fatness. We are often encouraged to eat more even when we're not hungry.

4. Women often have an inappropriate 'emotional' relationship with food. This causes us to eat for all the wrong reasons, building up bad eating habits.

5. Many dieters have low self-esteem – you have to value yourself if you want to lose weight, because you must believe you are worth investing in.

Now: what do you do next? The most important thing is to learn the principles behind the healthy eating. Having an understanding of why and what you eat will help you to take responsibility for your lifestyle.

The first thing to decide is: do you want to tiptoe or dive straight in to your new lifestyle?

You will lose weight automatically if you start to change your whole way of life and eating pattern to a 'healthy eating' regime. Adopting a new, healthy way of living will always make you lose weight and feel like a million dollars, no matter how lightly – or religiously – you apply the new outlook to your life. But (and this is a big BUT) the more tentative you are in implementing the changes, the slower the weight loss will be.

All weight-loss and fitness experts think that a slow, steady progress is best when it comes to losing weight. However – we live in a fast-moving world. And when you are fighting the battle of the bulge, you feel the need to see results faster than that. After all, we've got a lot of bad mistakes to undo – a lot of weight to lose that shouldn't be there. A loss of just a pound a week may not be enough to keep our spirits up, especially while we are making huge efforts to change our ways.

So, Jason has devised a special 21 day 'kick-up-the-bum' diet plan, based sensibly upon his healthy eating principles, which will give you a boost in your weight-loss plans. It is a sort of turbo-boosted version of the healthy eating lifestyle, based on the same health-giving, life-enhancing principles that you should eventually be applying to your whole diet. It's a crash course in healthy eating, but the backbone of the plan is something you can take with you for the rest of your life. In his description of the 21 Day Kickstart (see Appendix A), Jason talks about '21 days *and beyond*'. The kickstart plan will get you started on your new regime, but the lessons you are learning will be with you for life. Jason calls them 'Health Rules For Life' and these guidelines can be broken down as follows:

1. No white flour products whatsoever!

Jason goes into more detail about these kinds of foods later in the book, but you're basically looking to avoid anything made with white flour – so pizza, pasta, rice, bread and cakes, to name a few. Remember that wholemeal flour alternatives are generally available for all these white flour products though – so you don't have to give up sandwiches and spaghetti for all time, just make sure you are eating the healthy option! *Wholemeal flour products only*.

To help you understand why refined white flour products are out (because there is a reason behind every 'rule'): these products have been stripped of virtually all vitamins, minerals and fibre. White flour bread and pasta are also quickly converted into sugar once in the system. Without the vitamins, minerals and fibre (which all help to slow down the absorption of sugars in the bloodstream), blood sugar levels rise far too rapidly and cause an immediate imbalance. The pancreas then has no alternative but to produce the 'Fat Producing Hormone' insulin to burn off the excess sugar. This excess 'energy' then gets transported to the liver and muscles for short-term energy use – and the remainder gets shoved into fat cells! Many people who are overweight are not suffering from 'pig-ism' or 'greed-ism' (as most people who judge overweight people believe), but have something called 'hyperinsulinism', or 'Syndrome X'. This means that, due to these white flour products, the pancreas has been asked to do too much for too long – and is now malfunctioning. The result is that when refined sugar and carbs are consumed, the pancreas over-secretes insulin; this often leads to too much insulin being present in the bloodstream constantly. When this happens, not only does the insulin push the sugars directly into fat cells, it also prevents already stored fat from being broken down. This is why so many people find it hard to lose weight even when they eat less. The answer is not to eat *less* refined sugar and carbs, but to rectify the sugar imbalance by not eating them *at all*. Of all the health rules this is the most important on the food front. No white flour products whatsoever!

2. 70% 'live' foods daily

'Live' foods are what I describe as 'living foods': foods which haven't been 'refined' or had the majority of their nutrients removed. These include all raw fresh fruits, vegetables and natural nuts (not roasted and salted). It also includes all lightly cooked vegetables, such as steamed or stir fried broccoli, green beans, peppers, carrots and so on.

All 'living' foods have been virtually 'pre-digested' by the plant itself, and therefore require little or no energy to digest, assimilate and dispose of in the body. This frees up valuable energy which helps to shift toxins from the system – including the toxic waste stored in fat cells.

The remaining 30% of your diet in the 'New You Lifestyle' should ideally be made up of fresh fish, lean white meats and 'whole' carbohydrates – such as wholemeal bread, wholegrain rice and pasta and so on. Dairy products should be eaten sparingly and we suggest only 3–5% of your overall diet to be made up of them. Reduced fat spreads should be used in place of butter. Jason also recommends that, in the spirit of this emphasis on 'live' foods and healthy eating, you should cut right down on tea and coffee, and wean yourself off sugary, fizzy drinks – even if they are low-cal, they are still packed full of chemicals! Water or fresh juices (vegetable or fruit) are the best beverages for your new lifestyle.

3. Get veggie juiced every day!

One of the easiest ways to guarantee that you get your daily 70% quota of 'live' foods is to get juiced every day. When you put veggies through a juice extractor you are once again freeing up work for your system. The juice machine extracts the juice from the fibres to leave a liquid packed with 'live' nutrients which are absorbed into your system with ease. Veggie juices may sound awful, but once made in the right way they are heaven. Have a look at the delicious recipes in this book for some ideas (see Appendix C) or go to www.thejuicemaster.com.

4. Eat processed and refined foods in emergencies and 'when in Rome' moments only

All food is good – if you don't have a choice. If, for example, you're climbing Mount Everest, you will find that it's pretty tricky to make a juice or find fresh fruit and vegetables. In this case one of the best 'food' sources is high cocoa content chocolate! However, when you *do* have a choice, then this isn't the best food choice. Because we are dealing with the real world we realise there will be times when you are in a situation where there really won't be anything 'good' to eat. When this happens, and if you're genuinely hungry, do eat! Just do your best to keep to the New You Lifestyle Health Rules For Life – especially rule number five…

5. No carbohydrates after 6pm

This is explained in full in The Juice Master Guidelines in Appendix A. This 'rule for life' is one of the most important, especially if you're trying to lose weight *and* keep it off. The results of this one rule alone can be quite dramatic on the weight loss front!

6. Eat only when genuinely hungry

You cannot feed any emotion with food. If you try, it's highly likely that what you eat will be converted into fat. Before eating anything it's worth taking a minute to ask yourself if you really are hungry or just tired, bored or whatever. Food can *never* help any emotion; all it ends is that empty, insecure feeling called hunger. Follow the twenty minute rule: if you're still hungry twenty minutes after your first craving, then allow yourself a small, healthy snack.

7. Leave at least three hours in between main meals before eating anything

Your digestive system was never designed to constantly be at work and it is vital that you give it some rest. It takes an average of three hours for a meal to leave your stomach and move into the intestinal tract, which is why we have given this time frame. *This doesn't mean eat every three hours* (you should only eat when genuinely hungry), it just means that this is the shortest period between meals. By not picking in between meals you also get to experience the real pleasure in eating: ending a hunger. When you pick at food all the time a true hunger never gets time to build, so you end up missing out on the real pleasure of eating. When you have let a hunger build you will also find that food tastes so much nicer.

8. Have a 'Natural Day' one day every week

This is a superb health tool for life. A 'Natural Day' involves eating and drinking *only* natural 'live' foods. Fruits, vegetables, nuts and juices. Many people find this easiest on a Sunday, when you have more control over what you eat. This 'rule' is more of a guideline, but the benefits are tremendous.

9. MOVE – and avoid Furniture Disease! Aim to get two lots of 20 minute stints of 'till you sweat' exercise every day

'Furniture Disease' affects millions of people in this country and, other than what they eat, it is the single biggest cause of weight gain, heart disease, stress and 'no life'. Our bodies were designed to move – not to sit for hours and hours on various bits of furniture! Clearly in today's world many of us, because of our jobs, have little choice but to sit on various bits of furniture for many hours at a time. However, this doesn't mean we then need to come home and sit on more bits of furniture for the rest of the day's hours. There are 168 hours in a week, so if you spend a couple of hours down the gym, you are still spending 166 hours a week on furniture! The minimum you need to do – for real results – is two lots of 20 minute stints of 'till you sweat' exercise every day. If you're just starting out then you may need to build up to that level, but the key is to move when you can.

Music often inspires people and a good investment is a mini-disc player or a walkman. You can then record music which inspires you – it makes working out so much more pleasurable! A mini-trampoline is another great investment: it works every single muscle in the body, is easy on the joints and it's also a lot of fun.

10. 6–8 hours of sleep/rest daily

We are now in a world where it's almost a crime to feel tired! People try to avoid the body's genuine desire for rest by falsely stimulating the system with things like caffeine and nicotine. Sleep and rest are essential to good health – so turn off the TV and go to bed!

11. Never eat any cooked food three hours before you sleep

This is a very important health rule for the New You lifestyle. When you sleep your metabolism drastically slows down and so the digestion of food becomes difficult. This often leads to the food sitting in your stomach for many hours – leading to a 'food hangover' and that Monday morning feeling. It also means you're often not hungry in the morning, as your system is still dealing with last night's leftovers. If you make this a rule for life you will wake up brighter, more refreshed and with a good hunger, ready to be satisfied with some 'live' juices and fresh fruits.

12. Always have something exciting to look forward to

In life you tend to get what you focus on. Your thoughts literally shape your future. If you focus on 'FAT' you will remain 'FAT'; if you focus on 'slim' there's a huge chance you will become slim! Every day, take time to visualise the New You. Close your eyes and vividly see yourself as the New You you want to be. Visualise waking up feeling light and looking slim. See yourself wearing the clothes you will be wearing when you become the New You. As you have your eyes closed, smile: you know you're on your way and that you, like me, will get there in the end. Get excited as you see yourself with a slim, trim, energy driven body! Feel how good it feels to know that you will soon be living every day as a slim and healthy person. See yourself in a swimming costume on a beach, looking good and feeling great. By closing your eyes and seeing yourself as the New You, your brain will automatically move in that direction. This may seem like a strange thing to do at first, but it is very, very important and will make your journey even easier than it's already going to be. Once you arrive in the slim land of 'The New You", find something else to visualise and look forward to. Looking forward to something keeps us alive in every way.

Finally –

13. Always see foods as they really are

Our minds, like our taste buds, can easily be manipulated and there is no question that certain food companies have managed to manipulate our minds very successfully into seeing one thing when the reality is very different. It is important to start seeing foods as they really are and not what food companies want us to see. For example, when I see chocolate, I see something very different to most. Ever since we were born we have been conditioned to see chocolate as a catalyst to emotional bliss! The reality is of course the opposite. If you eat chocolate when you're feeling down, you don't all of a sudden feel good – in fact all that happens is you feel worse! When I see chocolate, I only see a load of white refined sugar, refined fat and chemicals – all covered in a gluelike substance which will stick to the walls of your intestines. The reason I see it as this is simply because this is precisely what it is. However, most people don't see this, as they've been conditioned to see it as the food company wants them to see it. The idea, with all foods, is to see them as they really are and not as 'they' want you to see them. Be free to make your own choices and see beyond the advertising, conditioning and brainwashing. Go back to basics, and eat the foods that Mother Nature intended – your body (and your figure) will thank you for it!

Getting Started

So, these are the principles of the New You lifestyle. But how can you put them into practice? There are basically two ways you can approach this. You can tip-toe warily into the water, or dive straight in. Alternatively, tiptoe at first, test the water, and once you have become used to it, dive in – with full confidence about what you are doing. Read on to find out more...

The tiptoe approach

This basically means that you learn and practise healthier living and eating, adopting the healthy lifestyle principles slowly but surely. This is how I did it: I studied the basic lessons of the 'Health Rules For Life' and then implemented them, one by one, into my new life. In other words, I did my homework first – I learned all the vital principles of eating *only* healthy foods, learning to turn my nose up at refined white breads, pastas, pizzas and rice: learning, understanding and believing why. I got into the habit of making morning juices and smoothies for breakfast, of opting only for wholemeal breads, pastas and brown rices, and of never touching carbohydrates after 6pm.

This took time. I practised this new, healthier way of eating – eating as much as I liked as long as the food was healthy – for more than a month.

I got up in the morning and first drank a glass of water. Then, after a bath or shower, I went downstairs and made myself a morning juice. If I was still hungry, I'd have a slice or two of wholemeal bread, with some fruit.

For elevenses, I'd have a glass of orange juice and a pitta bread, stuffed with tomato salad or some hummus with wholemeal bread.

For lunch I'd make myself a soup, and then a smoked salmon sandwich, bulking it out with lots of cucumber, celery and salad leaves. Or a baked potato with tuna salad.

For supper, I'd have a veggie stir fry or an avocado salad. If I was nibbly, I'd eat lots of dips with carrot and celery sticks.

The evenings, when I had been in the habit of eating tons of rice and pasta, were the only tough time. But I stuck at it – no carbs after six – and, in the end, it did get easier. Sometimes in the evenings, I would have a drink (yes I know that's a carbohydrate – aagh!) but I would make a real effort to stop at only one.

That's the main lesson of this healthy eating lifestyle – you can have as much as you want, as long as it is totally healthy food. No substitutes or alternatives. Back to nature. Eating food the way Mother Nature intended: that way your body will respond by losing weight if you need to, or maintaining a healthy weight for your body and lifestyle.

Honestly, you need do no more than that, and the results will – slowly but surely – speak for themselves.

Diving straight in

If you are desperate to lose weight, however, you may feel that the tiptoe approach is too slow. You're probably saying, 'OK, I understand that I have got to switch to totally healthy foods – but I want to lose weight faster…'

For people like you (and that's possibly most of us!), Jason has devised a special 21 Day Kickstart plan. It's exactly like the healthy eating lifestyle, and based entirely around its principles – but with added restrictions for quicker results. Embarking on the 21 day plan will still teach you everything you need to know – just as you go along. Follow it to the letter, and you will adopt a healthy eating regime as well as learning how to prepare nutritious, healthy food which you'll love for the rest of your life. And it's no mistake that it is designed for 21 days. Some scientists reckon that it takes just 21 days for the human brain to 'unlearn' old habits and pick up a new one. I personally think that it takes a lot longer than 21 days to kick the chocolate habit! But certainly, after 21 days, you will feel as though you have been detoxed, cleaned up, scrubbed from the inside out and set on a new road – and that's exactly what you want.

Tiptoeing and then diving

This was the way I did it. I learned the 'Health Rules For Life' until I could hear them in my sleep. Every time I got in the car to do the school run, I would play my 'retuning' CD until I knew every word. Every time I went to the shops, I could see the Health Rules For Life like a book page in front of my eyes, as I trudged up and down the supermarket aisles. Get those new ideas firmly into your brain, and then practise them. Try approaching every meal with a new idea. Instead of cooking white pasta, try brown wholemeal. If the kids turn up their noses at it, introduce it gradually – at first with just 25% wholemeal, then 50%. Make sandwiches with one side white and the other brown. And tell the family why you are doing it. Believe me, kids know more about nutrition than you think – they're beginning to be taught about it at school. Tell them how white pasta, bread and rice pushes up their blood sugar levels, and explain the harm that can do. Every time you explain it to others, you will be reinforcing the information in your own brain. You have to utterly believe it. I am sorry to keep repeating this – but it is truly what makes the difference between all those diets you're tried and failed, and a lifestyle change which will give you the long term results you want.

Once you have come to this stage, then if you want quicker weight loss, now is the time that you too can dive in: go for the 21 day plan. You'll find it much easier to do than someone who's approaching it anew – because it won't feel so strange and alien.

I was practising the 'Health Rules For Life' for nearly two months before I embarked on the 21 day plan – and wow, did I get results. I lost thirteen pounds in the first two weeks, and another three in the third week.

So, some points to remember – in a nutshell:

- You will lose weight just by eating healthily, following the Health Rules For Life from our lifestyle plan.

- To lose weight more quickly – after you have really practised the New You principles (I would recommend for at least a month) – try the 21 day plan.

- The 21 day plan is fully explained by Jason in Appendix A, and outlined with meal plans in Appendix B. It basically consists of:

  First two days: nothing but water, juices and smoothies.

  Days 3–5: water, juices, smoothies, raw fruits, raw veggies and salads with avocados or walnuts – still only raw, 'live' foods, but as much as you like. So, juice for breakfast, salads for lunch and smoothies for dinner.

  Days 6 and 7: everything as before but now with added yoghurts, and fruit-only smoothies.

  Days 8–21: everything as before, but with added carbohydrates and proteins – for instance, wholegrain sandwiches, stir fries, fish and chips and so on. So that's juices or smoothies for breakfast, carbohydrates for lunch and protein meals for dinner.

And if you think that sounds boring – then just take a look at the recipes which Jason suggests for each day (Appendix C). Mouthwatering or what?!

Let's just go over this again, because this *is* the path to success.

There are two ways you can lose the weight you want:

Route A: Learn the Health Rules For Life and apply them to your daily life from now on. You will slowly and surely learn new habits, and your body weight will gradually adjust. You will lose weight easily, but slowly.

Route B: Dive straight into the 21 day plan, which is a quick fire version of the Health Rules For Life, specifically designed for speedy weight loss. It is harder work and pretty restrictive, but it will teach you all the right eating principles, and give a boost to your new healthy eating lifestyle. After the 21 day plan, you simply switch to the lower gear and more permissive Health Rules For Life.

Or, of course, you can do what I did, and combine these paths – by following 'A' first for a month or two, and then doing 'B'. Remember that the 21 day plan is within a set time limit for a reason, too, so whenever you complete it make sure you relax back into the Health Rules For Life again. The kickstart is just that, and should only be followed for the allotted 21 days.

Amazing facts about our favourite fruits and veggies (just in case you're tempted to go back to a diet of rubbish!)

Did you know that restaurants sell more salads on Mondays than on any other day of the week? Did you know that more people go to fitness centres and gyms on Mondays than on any other day of the week?

The truth is – we all make 'New Year's Resolutions' every Sunday night – and they generally last until Tuesday lunchtime!

Let's all accept that our eating habits will never be perfect. But what about aiming for perfection 70, 80 or even 90% of the time? That way, you won't feel you've failed when you do grab a pot of noodles, or a chip butty. As Jason explains later in the book, it's what you do *most* of the time that matters.

So now arm yourself with the true, astonishing facts about Nature's best foods – and you'll find it easier to go for the healthy option.

- Eating fruits and vegetables reduces blood pressure, and thus decreases your risk of heart disease. Fibre, potassium, magnesium and calcium all reduce blood pressure, and are all found in fruits and vegetables.

- Eating a variety of fruits and vegetables reduces your risk of cancer. Folate, a vitamin found in citrus fruits, citrus juices and green leafy vegetables, is associated with the prevention of colon, rectal, cervical, lung, stomach and oesophageal cancers.

- Folate, vitamin B6 and vitamin B12 reduce your risk of heart disease, and may reduce your risk for colon cancer, Alzheimer's disease, miscarriages, birth defects, osteoporosis, strokes and ageing of the eyes.

- Eating a variety of fruits and vegetables provides your digestive tract with fibre. Fibre reduces constipation, diverticulosis, and your risk for cancer of the digestive tract and diabetes.

- Fruits and vegetables are needed to develop strong bones. Vitamin C, vitamin K, potassium and magnesium are necessary for bone regeneration and are all found in fruits and veggies.

There's a neat guide to the best sources of minerals and vitamins at the back of this book on pages 249–50, but here's a brief look at what some of my favourite veggies can do for us all:

ASPARAGUS Did you know, it's a member of the lily family, and related to onions, leeks, and garlic? So it's not surprising to hear that asparagus 'cleanses' the blood and is good for kidneys and bowels. It contains beta-carotene, vitamins B1 and C, bioflavinoids, potassium, and a special amino acid called aspargagine. Some say that this soothes a nervous mind. The taste of the juice is a little 'dry' so mix with strong fruity flavours like apple or carrot. I personally like asparagus lightly steamed, with lemon juice and black pepper!

BEETS Now these are famous for their ability to cleanse the blood. Beets contain calcium, sulphur, iron, potassium, choline, beta-carotene and vitamin C – and are also high in minerals which strengthen the liver and gall bladder. I've always liked pickled beetroot but you can also juice the raw, uncooked beets – mix them with carrot or apple. Beet juice is thought to be therapeutic in the treatment of leukemia and cancer.

BROCCOLI This is amazingly good for you. Broccoli is high in protein and fibre and is full of beta-carotene, vitamins B1 and C. It contains calcium, sulphur and potassium, as well as a substance called inderol-3 that emulsifies oestrogen, reducing the risk of breast cancer in women. Juice along with carrot or apple – or eat raw with dips!

BRUSSEL SPROUTS Like broccoli, they are a good source of vitamin C, potassium, calcium, sulphur, vitamin A, and 44% of the calories in brussel sprouts come from protein. Better eaten lightly cooked.

CABBAGE Don't cook this – chop it up raw and eat with salads! It's an excellent source of beta-carotene, sulphur, vitamin C and the trace mineral selenium, which is excellent for fighting cancer, protecting against heart disease, improving conditions of arthritis, slowing the ageing process, giving beautiful skin and increasing male potency. Within cabbage is a delicate amino acid called glutamine which is excellent for healing stomach disorders including ulcers.

CARROTS An 8oz glass of carrot juice contains 20,000 mg. of vitamin A – completely safe in the vegetable form. Vitamin A is an antioxidant that is able to attach to 'free radicals' (rogue molecules in the body which attack cells and tissues), stopping them in their tracks. The damaging effect of free radicals has been associated with cancer and, of course, ageing. Try a glass of carrot juice in the morning instead of coffee – it packs as much immediate punch, as its natural sugars are released very quickly. It also contains minerals, like organic calcium, as well as vitamins B and C, iron, potassium, phosphorus, and sodium. Vitamin A also helps your body fight infection, and keeps your skin and hair healthy. Carrot juice is also reputed to be a natural healer, good for the liver, intestines and nervous system.

CELERY A favourite ingredient for my morning juice! Its juice is reputed to be the best way to stop a headache and is said to be a superb nerve tonic. It also helps cure a craving for sweet things, cools you down if you are feeling the heat and is said to cleanse the body of carbon dioxide! High in magnesium, iron, chlorophyll and organic sodium (salt) – so great when added to soups and stocks, as you won't need to add any salt.

GARLIC There are entire books written about the curative abilities of garlic – reducing blood pressure, helping with the problems of blood clotting and cholesterol... It also boosts the immune system and helps recovering heart attack victims! Garlic's famous smell comes from allicin, which inhibits bacterial growth and fungus. It helps with an overgrowth of yeast in the body and is used in treating candida. Garlic also increases the flow of digestive enzymes and encourages detoxification through the skin. Throwing a clove of garlic in your veggie juice every day will be excellent for your health, but it may stop your friends coming around!

LETTUCE The leaves of any lettuce that is dark green in colour will be rich in chlorophyll and a good source of sulphur, chlorine, silicon and vitamin B – all contributing to hair growth, healthy skin and defences against lung cancer. Iceberg lettuce, though, has barely more to offer than a glass of water – but is nice and crispy in salads!

PARSLEY Parsley is effective for upset stomachs by stimulating digestive enzymes. It is also excellent for the colon. Parsley is good to add to veggie juices because it is high in chlorophyll, which acts like iron to oxidise the blood.

POTATOES They are in the same family as tomatoes and peppers. An excellent source of vitamin C and high in carbohydrates, potassium, calcium and iron. The most nutritious part of the potato is the skin.

SPINACH Another good veg to add to juices because it is so high in chlorophyll as well as nutrients such as oxalic acid, beneficial in the cleansing and healing of the intestinal tract. Cooking destroys all the best qualities, so juice it – ensuring you mix it with sweeter, lighter juices like apple, pineapple and celery – or chop it up raw into salads.

And now the fruits:

TOMATOES Yes, a tomato is a fruit, not a vegetable. Packed with vitamin C, one tomato gives us 80% of the vitamin C we need each day for healthy gums, muscles and skin. Tomatoes are also good for sodium phosphorus, calcium, potassium, magnesium, malic and oxalic acids and sulphur. Fresh tomato juice has a wonderful taste that is quite different from the store-bought juice which is boiled and stored in cans for months.

BERRIES Blackberries, blackcurrants, redcurrants, raspberries, strawberries, gooseberries and bilberries are all brilliantly good for you as they all contain large concentrations of phytochemicals. The darker the fruit, the more phytochemicals it has and the more nutritious it is. These phytochemicals are thought to have lots of beneficial properties: some are anti-bacterial, some anti-inflammatory, some protective against cancer, and others may help to reduce cholesterol. Most phytochemicals are also antioxidants.

CHERRIES The same chemicals that give tart cherries their colour may relieve pain better than aspirin and ibuprofen in humans, so eating about 20 tart cherries a day could reduce inflammatory and headache pain.

BANANAS My all time favourite food, eaten raw, blended into smoothies, baked on a barbie or even simply mashed into a sandwich! Did you know that it's not actually a fruit – it's a herb, and there are over 500 different types of banana in the world? Bananas are about 99.5% fat free. Bananas are a great source of potassium, which helps build muscle power and keeps your body fluids in balance.

But let me end on the humble **APPLE** – a continuing favourite for almost everyone, handy in juices, a brilliant snack, bursting with nutrients, high in phytochemicals, antioxidants, vitamins and fibre. Apples contain a natural antiseptic (malic acid) that helps keep your breath fresh. No wonder they say an apple a day keeps the doctor away! And did you know that fresh apples will float because 25% of their volume is air?

chapter 5

the new you lifestyle

So, what comes next? Well, it's your life, so you are free to choose the recipes and meals which suit your lifestyle best. Here's what I do now, after completing the 21 day plan and starting out on my own. This is an idea of my new, healthy lifestyle – and it really does work!

Breakfast time

First – wake up, yawn and drink a glass of water. That will help rehydrate you after a night's sleep, and will wash your system through.

Next – you should get moving! Do something to wake up your body. I have been going downstairs and doing five minutes' bouncing on the trampoline in the garden. Make yourself do a five minute routine every morning, before you even think about it! It doesn't have to be trampolining, you can run up and down the stairs energetically, pop an exercise video on and do a quick morning workout, or take the dog for a very brisk walk around the block.

Then you want to get some quick and easy vitamins and nutrients inside your body, so make yourself a juice, or a fruit smoothie. That just means chopping up a few of your favourite fruits and veggies, bunging them in a juicer, blending them with some ice and maybe an avocado – and drinking! It's refreshing and it is jam packed with nutrients. Like taking a tonic – only tasty!

Why juice?

Let's get this straight. Probably nothing is better for you than eating fruits and vegetables. In a juice, you can drink in all of the nutrients from lots of different fruits and veg far more quickly than you could eat them whole. You can include veggies in your breakfast juice – like celery, cucumber, peppers – which you would never normally eat in the morning.

Why is that important?

Well, you don't want to drink only fruit juice, because it is too high in sugar (even though it's natural sugar) if you are trying to lose weight. Even an abundance of natural sugars, juiced from apples, oranges, pineapples and strawberries, would spike your blood sugar levels – and this is what you want to avoid from now on. Adding veggie juices helps dilute the effect.

The goal is to keep your blood sugar at an even keel, no great highs or lows. Remember that, if your blood sugar level goes up and down too extremely, your body produces insulin to balance things out, and this results in your body storing the excess sugar as body fat.

The only drawback of juicing is the washing up afterwards. Juicers are a nuisance to wash! I used to be very good and wash mine up straight away – before I even drank the juice. Nowadays, I juice before everyone else has breakfast, and then put the used parts into the sink with all the other breakfast things!

If you can't juice, then blend yourself a smoothie. Try to include some veggies in the mix – but it's not quite so important for your blood sugar levels, because you will be eating all the fibre from the fruit too, unlike in a straight juice, and that will help your body to digest the mix slowly, thus avoiding sugar highs. Try adding either an avocado or a banana for bulk; these are rich in natural oils and beneficial nutrients.

It's the same with eating the fruit whole. Because you are absorbing all of the fruit, you are eating it as Nature intended – and digesting all that fibre and pulp helps your body digest slowly. Your blood sugar level won't spike.

So that's breakfast: you will find, especially if you make yourself busy, that a juice or smoothie is surprisingly filling and will keep you going until lunchtime. If you really are beginning to wilt before then (and remember from now on, you only want to eat if you are really hungry), then have what you want as a mid morning snack. Remember, it's fine as long as it is healthy, whole food. Jason has put together a whole list of tasty snacks to give you some ideas – check out his suggestions on pages 241–5.

The main thing to remember here is that, while your habits may be telling you that you want a couple of biscuits or a slice of cake – they are just habits. They are not what your body needs, and now they are not what your brain wants either. Try to develop a habit for eating something else. You will find that, if you persevere, you will develop a real taste for something far healthier.

Lunchtime

Again, there are no rules except eating only when you are hungry and eating healthy, whole foods.

I like a Caesar salad (if you're not a vegetarian, you can add chicken) or a Salad Nicoise (tuna and beans). If you are really hungry in these early days then have salad and a soup – made at home with basic, whole ingredients. Again, you can accompany this with rye or seeded breads. But it doesn't have to be a salad – you could make yourself a quick and easy stir-fry (use virgin olive oil) with wholegrain rice. Or what about a baked jacket potato with tuna or egg, sweetcorn and crème fraiche?

Again, if you are hungry (*really* hungry!) mid-afternoon, you can eat whatever you really want for a snack. I preferred rice cakes, pitta bread and some fruit.

Dinnertime

Again, you eat what you really want. I loved a grilled swordfish or salmon steak with stir-fried vegetables. Perhaps you would prefer a tasty bit of steak with salad? Get used to eating fruit for dessert – or a little cheese with celery. There's actually nothing wrong with strawberries and cream. If it is healthy, natural food, then it's yours. But let's be sensible. Although there is nothing wrong with butter, cream and mayonnaise – and do remember to eat them sparingly – you *are* trying to lose weight. Only on the Atkins diet can you eat as much of those high-fat ingredients as you like… and I personally worry about that diet, don't you? In this new, healthy-eating lifestyle change, we want to adopt a new attitude towards food, and thinking you can glut out on high fat foods and full fat dairy products is a mistake – and no way towards a healthy eating pattern for the future.

And what to drink? Well, one thing you should remember is water, water, water. It takes time, but you really can develop a taste for it! If you are lucky and live in one of those areas of Britain which has good-tasting tap water, then just opt for that – big glasses of it, spruced up with ice and a wedge of lemon or lime.

Otherwise, experiment with a water filter to see if the taste improves. Of course, you can buy bottled water, but with the amount you should be drinking (at least eight large glasses a day) your wallet will soon feel the pinch.

I like water with the tiniest drop of fruit juice in it (again, it's amazing how quickly you get used to it!), with ice and a sprig of mint. Have a go at making your own water cocktails!

Fruit juices on their own can be high in sugar – albeit natural sugar. Fizzy and diet drinks can be loaded with additives. You have to ask yourself if that is really what you want to be drinking nowadays anyway.

When I gave up drinking diet cola, I actually suffered from a headache for a day or two – but now I feel much better, and richer!

And now the sixty million dollar question – should you drink alcohol?

The short answer is – it depends how quickly you want to lose weight. Although alcohol doesn't contain any fat, it *is* high in calories and it can also cause a sugar high – just as refined and processed carbohydrates can. Alcohol is also an appetite stimulant so, if you are not careful, you will think you are hungry, when you are not!

It's up to you. It may well be that alcohol in moderation is one of those old habits you would like to keep. At least occasionally!

But while you are really, really trying to lose weight – don't! It ain't worth it – unless you absolutely know you can stop at *one*, and it won't trigger a binge or a nibble. Remember to ask yourself – why is it so important to you to have alcohol? Are you emotionally drinking? Are you drinking out of mere habit? If it's a 'kick' you are after, what about the 'kick' you'll get from being slim and fit? Which is more desirable?

During the months when I really wanted to lose weight fast, I stopped drinking alcohol altogether. Nowadays, I just have one occasionally. At drinks parties, I can quite happily sip at a mineral water or fruit juice. The pressure to join in with others is really only in your head.

Note that I keep saying: 'eat what you want if you are *really* hungry', or 'have it if you *really* want'. I am emphasising the 'really' as a way of reminding you to ask yourself this very question.

When you are tempted to have biscuits and cakes, ask yourself – with everything you now know about the nature of processed refined foods and what they do to your body – 'do I *really* want this?'

When you walk into the kitchen to prepare yourself some food without thinking, ask yourself – with what you really know about habits – 'am I *really* hungry?'

When you feel fed up, bored or miserable and find yourself sitting down with a packet of biscuits, ask yourself – 'with all I now know about emotional eating, will eating this *really* make me feel better?'

Again, this is a habit that you can develop, and it *really* helps! I found that, even on days when I was unsure how I wanted to answer, I made a little pact with myself. I would put things off for 20 minutes. I thought – if I still want to eat this in 20 minutes time, then I will. But I'll do something else first. Usually, that would solve the problem.

This is also where visualisation can help enormously. At those times when you feel the full force of habit, are feeling low or craving a food – when you feel that, dammit, you *deserve* a slice of cake, you also need to bring all your determination back into focus by visualising how it will feel, how you will look when you are slim and fit.

If you have an old photo of yourself slim and healthy, then pin it up somewhere. If you have seen a particular outfit in a women's magazine, then cut it out and pin that up. Maybe even cut out a photo of your face and stick it on a slim body. Find yourself an image you can aspire to. Don't just look at it and sigh. Imagine it is you. Feel how good it is to be slim, how those clothes feel on your body. Love yourself in it. Spend a couple of minutes staring at the picture, then close your eyes and imagine that's how you are – now!

OK, I know it sounds a bit New Age, Californian, psycho-babble-ish. But that's visualisation. It's what all the modern athletes do – and they swear it makes the difference between winning and losing.

After all, it's exactly what a hypnotist would do with you.

I tried hypnotherapy for a while and used it as a way of reinforcing everything I'd learnt and reminding me of the way I *really* want to go! Hypnotists are expensive and you have to go back for many sessions. But what I found really useful was to make my own re-tuning CD which works on the same principles as hypnotherapy sessions, so that you can listen, over and over again, to the most important messages from this book.

It really helps. I know, because I used to listen to my re-tuning CD every time I got into the car. It is one of the things that made the difference. It's one of the things that helped me 'believe' in what I was doing.

It's almost like wide-awake, active hypnotism – I would find myself driving along, laughing, moaning, it's a mental 'top-up' of all the advice I already know – but listening to it repeatedly helps to drive it right inside the brain.

You can, of course, make your own CD or tape. Write yourself a script – just jot down all the ideas you have which you think might help you stay on track. As you read this book, highlight some of the points which especially ring true with you, and then just read them out to a tape recorder. Don't worry about how it sounds – no one is going to listen to it save yourself – but be careful not to leave it lying around! Then simply play it to yourself when you are on your own – that's why I always played it in the car, on the way to collect the kids from school, or on the way to the shops.

Talking of making tapes, you should also record some of your favourite music tracks for exercising to. I'll bet there are some songs that always cheer you up, always get you singing or smiling. If you put them on a special tape, and play them while you do your morning exercises, you will feel doubly refreshed. Research shows that people who exercise to music get a better body workout than those who exercise while watching the TV, or contemplating their own navel. Goodness knows how anyone gauged and measured that one – but clearly the brighter you feel, the greater the benefit!

(OK, now here's a confession. My first track is Elvis singing 'All Shook Up' followed by Joni Mitchell singing 'Carey' and then Gabrielle singing 'Sunshine'. Next, I have a bit of Mozart for the soul: 'Eine Kleine Nachtmusik', neatly rounded off with Queen and 'Bohemian Rhapsody'! By the time I've got through that one – I'm raring to go!)

Treat your body as though it belonged to your children, or your loved one. It is theirs, in a way, because the healthier you are, the greater your chances of living a long and healthy life with those you love.

Feed it with only the best, pamper it, exercise and tone it – gently at first, so that you learn to love your new lifestyle.

You will lose weight and feel better almost instantly – though it will not be like a crash diet, you will not lose masses of weight quickly. But it is a plan for life, and you will *never* put that weight on again.

Juicing

Drinking homemade, freshly squeezed juices is like absorbing liquid sunshine. It feels great, tastes delicious – and you are pouring into your body an express delivery of vitamins, minerals and other nutrients. It is the best, healthiest way to start the day.

It is the 'ultimate fast food' – because no way could I eat raw three whole apples, half a pineapple, five sticks of celery, a yellow pepper and half a cucumber for breakfast!

But, juiced into a glass, I can benefit from all their healthy, life-giving ingredients… all in one go.

Remember, you don't need a juicer to eat healthily. You don't have to have a juicer to follow this new healthy lifestyle (although it will help, particularly if you plan to follow the 21 Day Kickstart plan). There's nothing better for you than fresh fruit and vegetables, eaten whole, and juicing should not replace those whole fruits in your diet.

But sometimes it can be difficult to digest a plateful of fruit and especially veggies in the morning. Who wants a red pepper, parsnip or beetroot for breakfast? I don't!

Drinking homemade juices offers positive health benefits. Not only do you avoid the vitamin and mineral losses that can occur during cooking, you are also able to obtain a concentrated source of the antioxidant vitamins A, C and E, which mop up excess 'free radicals', the rogue molecules that attack cells and tissues and are linked with heart disease and some cancers.

While a medium-sized whole orange has around 85mg of vitamin C, a 200ml glass of freshly juiced orange can contain three times that amount. Juicing also breaks down the hard cell walls of fruits and vegetables, freeing the beta-carotene and making this nutrient easier to absorb.

You can use almost any raw fruit or vegetable in home juicers. While some juices, especially those made from green vegetables, can be an acquired taste, apple, carrot, parsnip, red pepper and citrus fruit juices tend to be instant favourites. Carrots and apples, in particular, have sweet flavours that blend very well with other juices. Remember to include veggies in your juice: this will keep your blood sugar levels low. As you know, the natural sugars in fruit juices can cause a blood sugar rise, so even things out by including celery (a cool flavour), cucumber (even cooler!), or perhaps yellow pepper (tangy). And then experiment!

Believe me, if you can acquire the taste, drinking juices every day will have an amazing effect on your skin, your energy levels and your whole body.

Please don't just think you can get the same benefits from shop-bought juices – even those in health food stores. Those juices were made weeks, if not months ago, and they taste nothing like the juices you can make at home.

The key to healthy, good-tasting juices is to experiment – but try not to mix more than two or three ingredients, otherwise you're likely to end up with a bit of a non-identifiable mush, with no main flavour coming through.

Of course, you can also take your juices and mix them with other fruits like bananas or avocados in your blender to make smoothies. A smoothie is a combination of whole soft fruits and either milk, yogurt or fruit juice, blended together with ice. You can use frozen fruits, too, like raspberries and blueberries. Just pop them straight into the blender from the freezer, along with any other fresh fruit and veggies you want, and maybe a little water. Keep the mix thick, and it's like a fruit sorbet, or ice cream. Yum!

Remember that even if you are becoming an avid juicer, you still need to drink lots of water. Try to stick to your eight glasses a day.

For more wonderful juice and smoothie ideas, please see Jason's delicious recipes on pages 208–18.

Two essentials to life – oxygen and water

You can't live for a moment without oxygen. You can't live for more than a couple of days without water. They're the two vital ingredients to living.

But do you know what? You might not be breathing or drinking appropriately! Even those functions might have to change as part of your new healthy lifestyle!

OK, I know that sounds odd. But it's a fact that most of us do not actually breathe as well – as deeply – as we could. We all breathe too shallowly nowadays – ask any singing teacher! It is also because we don't exercise enough – and you need a good pant to get that air to the bottom of your lungs!

So try adding a breathing routine to your morning workout – spend one or two minutes (to a favourite music track) doing deep breathing, arcing your arms above your head and down to your hips – just like those gym teachers taught us at school!

It's also a fact that most of us do not drink enough water – not nearly enough. We have become used to eating plenty (just look at the obesity rates) but drinking water is a forgotten art. How much water do you drink – really?

We should all be drinking at least eight tall glasses of water a day. However, the overweight person needs one additional glass for every 25 pounds (almost two stones) of excess weight. If you exercise briskly or if the weather is hot and dry, the amount you drink should also be increased. Not many of us drink enough. Yet it is crucial to running our bodies properly. As you have to have water in a car's engine (or it overheats and blows up), you need to be tanked up, too.

Water is an essential part of our bodily needs: it makes up approximately 55–65% of an adult's body weight. In fact, the body will also retain extra water if it isn't getting enough. That's why a great many women suffer from water retention. Some women are carting around an extra five or six pounds of water in the form of uncomfortable swollen ankles, knees and wrists – because they are overweight and not drinking enough. The best way to treat that problem is to drink more – pure water. Our metabolism depends on water to run efficiently – so give it what it needs.

One extra thought. Apparently we often eat more than we need, because we mistake thirst for hunger. So listen to your body and give it lots of water – it's actually more important than food – as it's what your body is crying out for!

Remember:

1. The rate at which we burn food or fat (our metabolism) is a chemical process requiring water. We need adequate water to ensure the smooth functioning of this process.

2. Water helps to flush toxins out of our system. The more toxins in our body, the less capable it is of functioning efficiently.

3. Water helps to prevent constipation. It's obvious, isn't it? You'll get clogged up without enough moisture!

4. Drinking lots of water gives you silky smooth and plump skin. It really does. My mother has always, for as long as I can remember, been a keen water drinker. Before she goes to bed, when she wakes up in the morning, at every meal and always just before she goes out anywhere. There you are, with the car's engine humming, waiting for her – and at the last moment, she always has to pop back into the kitchen for a drink of water. She is blah-blah years old (I am sorry, she won't let me say!) but her skin is supersmooth, like a child's. I just hope my kids will be able to say the same about me in years to come!

chapter 6

exercising for fun

I think what I liked about Jason was that he answered so many questions that had been nagging me for years. And one of the most compelling things about him was that he had been there himself – he had been fat and unfit, and he had turned his life around just by embracing a style of eating that was down to earth, sensible and fun.

'Are you fit?' he asked me, over that first glass of juice in our friend's kitchen.

Am I hell, I thought. But, 'I used to be!' I offered.

It's true. A couple of years ago, I had tried to lose weight by doing lots and lots (and lots!) of exercise. I was doing breakfast radio at the time – co-presenting LBC Breakfast in London every morning with Sir Nick Lloyd, former editor of the *Daily Express*, and husband of Eve Pollard (who, of course, used to be editor of the *Sunday Express*, and was at *TV-am* as Features Editor!).

I seem to be destined to present programmes with someone called Nick. Nick Lloyd and I got on like a house on fire. He was a true blue Tory – I was a sometime Green Party voter and a bit of a liberal – and it was election time, with John Major heading, inevitably, for defeat.

In the middle of everything, my divorce happened, in a blaze of horrendous publicity. The press (yet again!) surprised me at my front door, at three in the morning, and snapped some revolting photos. Needless to say, I was not looking my best – and so they were happy to point out that my husband might be leaving me because I had 'let myself go'.

Whilst my appearance wasn't my first concern, some weeks later, I decided to spruce myself up a bit and lose some weight. There was a gym in LBC right on the basement floor, about three doors away from our studio, and so I found it quite easy to pop in there almost every day, after my programme ended at 9am, and work with a brilliant trainer called Kate.

Later, a group of us would get together nearly every morning, and work through a very active and energetic routine with Roy, who used to be in the eighties dance troupe Hot Gossip. It felt brilliant, being that fit. I constantly astounded myself with my level of energy and enthusiasm. I even made an exercise video. When I look back on it now, I realise that I could never have committed to such a gruelling routine if I hadn't been in the extraordinary position of having a job which finished at 9am! On top of that, my children were still quite small, and their routines were fairly straightforward. I couldn't possibly put in that many hours nowadays. I am lucky if I can find an hour a day to exercise at home.

I lost a lot of weight, very successfully – and the video was a bestseller.

To celebrate its success, we all went out for dinner. And that was that. I stopped putting in those hours of exercise every day – and suddenly the weight started to pile on again.

Making that video certainly taught me that it feels good to be fit. But putting on the weight so quickly afterwards also taught me that, through all those months of concentrating on fitness, I had learned nothing about the core problem.

What was making me fat in the first place? While I worried about it, and became more and more miserable about my size, I just got bigger. I don't understand it, I thought. I eat healthy food. I am a vegetarian! I don't drink very much. I don't even crave chocolates and cakes, like some of my friends. Surely there could be nothing wrong with my eating habits?

And that question nagged away at me, so when Jason sat there in the kitchen, smiled at me with a frothy moustache of veggie juice, and asked me if I was fit, I had to be honest.

'I have hardly done any exercise at all for months,' I whispered, almost ashamed. 'It's even difficult getting up and out of bed in the morning. Every joint aches. I don't think my body fully wakes up until about ten past three in the afternoon!'

Just recently my back had been playing up, too. Some mornings, the small of my back was so painful that I could hardly make it to the bathroom – and pulling on a pair of trousers, or tights, was agonising! It could be like that all day – and then quite suddenly feel much better at about seven in the evening, when the day was already wasted. I felt like an old lady.

I used to like exercise, I used to actually get a buzz after a session in the gym, but the truth is that, once you have stopped exercising, once you have got out of the habit, the very thought of ever getting that fit again – well, it's exhausting just thinking about it! I just wish I had never let it go.

Several months before, I had dragged my old exercise bike out of the garage, brushed the cobwebs off it, and pulled it indoors for a quick ride. It had returned the favour by leaking filthy black oil spots all over the carpet. Then my eldest son took it apart, put it back together again and it gave up the ghost. After that, we hauled it out to the council dump. Maybe that's what had done my back in...

Getting some sort of exercise into my daily routine was so hard, that when Jason suggested trampolining to wake me up, well, I'd thought I'd go for it.

Now, I have got a very small garden – just enough room for a gin and tonic on the patio and a patch of lawn. Where on earth could I put a trampoline? Did I have enough room, or would one bounce land me in the neighbour's goldfish pond?

Being me, either greedy or over-exuberant with a new idea, I didn't just want a little trampet (although I now realise that that would have been fine!), I wanted a proper big one, on which we could all bounce as one happy, bouncing family.

The man from SuperTramps came around, and sized up the garden. 'Yes,' he said, 'We'll get one in here… You might not get it out again, but…'

So they came the following week, and erected a family-size, big, green bouncing machine on the lawn. And I had to fight the kids off, just to see if I really could do it.

Well, I have to tell you! If you are unfit, five minutes solid bouncing on a trampoline isn't just exhausting – it's knackering! But fun.

So nowadays, my early mornings start (unless it is pouring) with a five minute session on the trampoline – and it's a very good way of finding out what your neighbours get up to so early in the morning, I can tell you.

So anything that gets you moving has to be good. If trampolining takes your fancy but your budget doesn't stretch to a family-size one, then a mini one will work just as well. Exercise every part of your body: bounce not just on your feet, try sitting on it, with your feet on the ground and your bum on the trampet. Twenty bounces up and down every morning and you'll soon remember where your stomach muscles used to be!

Facing the demon – how to tackle the exercise issue

First things first – please remember that, just a few months ago, I hated the very idea of doing exercise. I felt quite depressed at the thought of pulling on an old T-shirt and jogging pants, and trudging down to my local gym. And yet, only a matter of weeks later, I had got to the point where I really did enjoy it.

I now feel better just walking up the road, just going up stairs, because I have now got muscles!

It's a brilliant sensation. If it can happen to me, it really can to you, too.

So I'm sorry to say it if you hate the idea right now, but if you're trying to lose weight, exercise is absolutely vital.

It needn't be as bad as it sounds. And you can start gently, gradually building up to a really exciting level of fitness. First you have to find something you like doing. Some people love to don their tracksuit, trainers and sweatband and go out jogging. I tried it and hated it – but I did find that I enjoyed cycling, both in a gym (while watching *Bewitched* on Channel 4 in the morning) and outside on a real bike with my sons pedalling alongside me. Some people love the atmosphere of gyms or aerobic classes, others opt for doing an exercise video at home, or skipping (or, in my case, trampolining) in the back garden. One tip, though, for prolonged success: it's often better to exercise with a friend, your partner or children, as you can get lonely on your own and on an off-day (and we all have them – even professional athletes) it's too easy to give up.

If you really want something unusual – how about learning to do 'Strip Aerobics'? Or bellydancing? Both are apparently very demanding activities and are efficient fat-burners! They're available on video now – which you can borrow from your local library – so if that's your thing, you've got no excuse!

Next, don't think you have to spend hours training. Like learning anything new, start with just ten minutes a day. But make it *every* day – and I guarantee you that within a week, you'll notice that it's becoming easier and you could go for longer.

Even a small amount of exercise will speed up your weight loss and keep you fit and healthy. And think of this – if you want to lose weight and you are not active, you'll need to eat 500 calories less per day than a slimmer who is doing exercise. Or to put it the other way around, you can eat more and still lose weight, provided you are exercising.

It may sound too simple to be true, but the easiest, cheapest and most sensible way for us all to get fitter is to walk. Thirty minutes of walking a day is a good initial target, or you could break it up into two 15 minute sessions. Walking is an injury-free way for the over-50s to keep fit, and kids are fitter when all the family walks together. Walk as though you are in a hurry, and swing your arms as you go. Wear a comfortable pair of trainers. You can't just loll along, though. The walking must be brisk. You know what I mean; you do have to feel a bit pink and sweaty afterwards.

Brisk walking burns off around 180 calories every 30 minutes. You will burn stored fat as fuel after the first 20 minutes. And the longer you walk, the more fat you will burn.

Daily exercising, however you do it, will help you to build up your metabolic rate if you have been very inactive, so that you use up more calories even when you are resting. It'll make you feel better by improving your mood and providing a sense of achievement and satisfaction. Aerobic activity – that is activity which exercises the heart muscle – burns calories, improves muscle tone and strength, relieves stress, and can also help with back pain, osteoporosis, respiratory problems, diabetes, arthritis, cardiac rehabilitation and a variety of other health problems. What have you got to lose?

You can count other things as exercise, too. Thirty minutes of brisk walking roughly equals:

- 45 minutes of house cleaning
- 20 minutes of a good aerobic workout
- 30 minutes cycling
- 40 minutes busy gardening
- 30 minutes shopping with heavy bags
- And don't forget swimming – half an hour of strenuous swimming is one of the best aerobic activities you can do.

So set yourself this goal: you are going to build exercise into your daily routine. It has to become a habit. Try keeping a chart each week to plan ahead and record how much progress you've made. But remember you've got to:

- make exercise fun
- don't be put off by a bad day – get over it and get back on track straight away!
- share exercise with friends
- build up slowly and think about how much you have achieved.

Finally, you probably hate exercising now *because* you are unfit. You will find that, as you become a little fitter, you will really enjoy the feeling. In fact, there is a chemical change going on inside you – your body starts to pump endorphins, which are natural chemicals designed to make you feel good.

Fitness experts are now recommending that one of the most efficient ways to lose fat is to do weight training to build muscle. Every pound of muscle burns 50 calories a day just by being there. So it makes sense that, the more muscle you have, the more fat you will burn, even when you are asleep.

Now this doesn't mean you have to have triceps like Arnold Schwarzenegger. Most of us have very little muscle – and it would do us all good to build them a little – not so they show as bulging muscle, just as firm flesh. That's why so many Hollywood actresses do weight training – it actually means they can stay fashionably emaciated without having to starve themselves.

Weight training is easy, you'll be glad to hear. You don't even need weights, and you don't have to spend very long doing it – just a few minutes a day.

Last summer, I met a gorgeous young American who has just recently made it big on TV in the States promoting a fitness regime he calls 'Eight Minutes In The Morning'. He's called Jorge (pronounced Hor-Hay) Cruise – and he's been tipped for the top by no less an admirer than Oprah Winfrey!

He reckons that all it takes is eight minutes of your time every day (he thinks first thing in the morning is best) to do a few easy exercises that will tone and build muscle throughout your whole body – and so fire your metabolism and promote weight loss.

His book outlines a month-long plan, where you complete a different set of exercises every day – it's all mapped out for you – until, by the end of the month, you have toned the whole body. Then you just keep repeating it, over and over.

Jorge says you can lose two pounds a week, if you combine this simple approach to weight training with a sensible, healthy diet. You'll build five pounds of muscle over a year. As a pound of muscle burns 50 calories a day – just by being there – that means you will automatically burn an extra 250 calories a day or 91,250 calories over a year. That's 26 pounds (or just under two stones in weight) in one year.

Astounding, isn't it?

I predict young Jorge will go far with that one – and I wish him luck. Details of his book are in the back of this one. I think it will be a great hit with millions of busy women – and especially those who hate gyms and aerobic classes. But can it really be that easy?

Well, all the experts are now recommending weight training, instead of, or as well as 15 or 20 minutes per day of aerobic exercise. Another book which I heartily recommend is *Strong Women Stay Young* by Miriam E. Nelson – possibly the first fitness expert to suggest that women can improve their whole body, and their health, by simple weight training. There are lots of exercise ideas in that one, too – and it discusses lots of special female issues like osteoporosis, the menopause and HRT (which are also dealt with in Chapter 11 of this book).

So, it looks like weight training is the new black – and here are some reasons for us all to follow the trend!

Eighteen reasons to do weight training

1. Weight training tones your muscles, which looks great and also raises your base metabolic rate, causing you to burn more calories 24 hours a day. You'll even burn more calories while you're sleeping!

2. Weight training can 'reverse' the natural decline in your metabolism which begins around age 30

3. Weight training energises you

4. Weight training has a positive effect on almost all of your 650-plus muscles

5. Weight training strengthens your bones, reducing your risk of developing osteoporosis

6. Weight training improves your muscular endurance

7. Weight training will NOT develop big muscles on women... just toned muscles!

8. Weight training makes you strong. Strength gives you confidence and makes daily activities easier

9. Weight training makes you less prone to low-back injuries

10. Weight training decreases your resting blood pressure

11. Weight training decreases your risk of developing adult onset diabetes

12. Weight training decreases your 'gastrointestinal transit time', reducing your risk for developing colon cancer

13. Weight training increases your blood level of HDL cholesterol (the good type)

14. Weight training improves your posture

15. Weight training improves the functioning of your immune system

16. Weight training lowers your resting heart rate, a sign of a more efficient heart

17. Weight training improves your balance and coordination

18. Weight training elevates your mood, making you feel more happy about yourself.

Fitness for the family

We all know that exercising on your own is not much fun – you get far more out of it if you can find an exercise buddy, to share your moans with but also to compete against.

Well, since you are no doubt the family cheerleader, how about roping the rest of the family into a new health and fitness regime?

Only, don't call it that, for goodness' sake. There's nothing like the words 'gym', 'fitness' or 'regime' to send them all screaming back to their bedrooms, armed with Game Boys and computer laptops.

When I first started heading for the gym in the evenings, I just casually asked my teenage sons if they'd like to come too.

Clearly, nothing was more abhorrent to them than going to the gym. Oh yes, there was something even worse: going to the gym with Mum.

So I said nothing more, and went on for the next few weeks, going alone.

I then, quite casually, asked them again.

Their first reaction was a firm no. But, by the time I had been upstairs to my

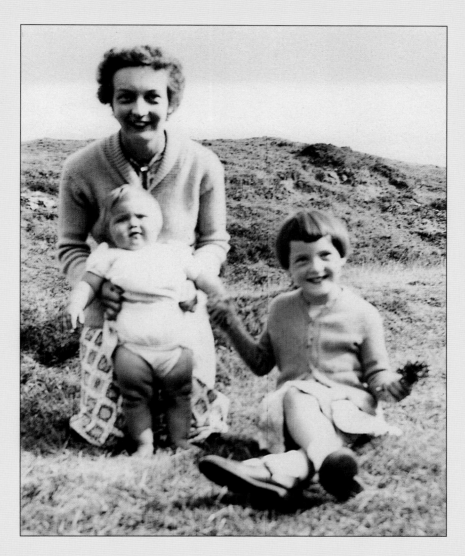

When I was a baby, my mother used to put an extra spoonful of formula into my milk. In post-war Britain, it was a matter of pride that mothers had "bonny" babies. My mum says she was always very proud of my sturdy legs, which are very much in evidence here! Shame I never shared her feelings, isn't it?!

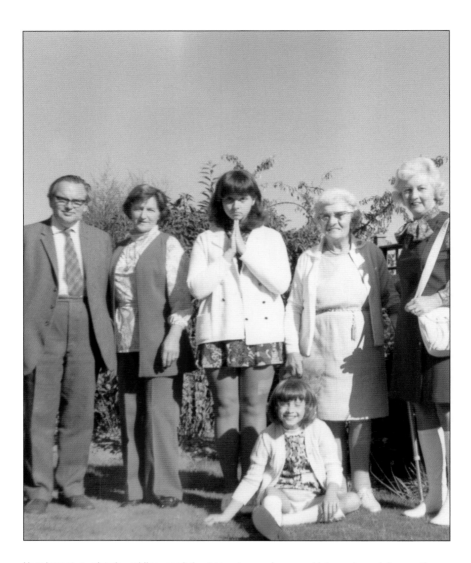

Here I am at my sister's wedding, aged about seventeen and squeezed into a micro mini as per the fashions of the time. I was so embarrassed about my legs when we got the pictures back! Even at that young age, I was already self-conscious about my figure and heavily critical of the way I looked.

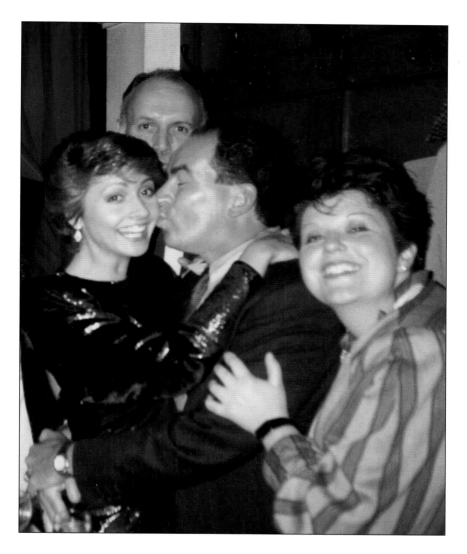

This is me on the night I presented Miss World. You cannot see much of me in this shot, but I had slimmed down to a minuscule size eight – mainly because of my worry about being compared to the contestants. My shimmering velvet dress was made specially for me by Bruce Oldfield: I have never been able to fit into it since that night! My best mate, Shirley-Anne, is at the front.

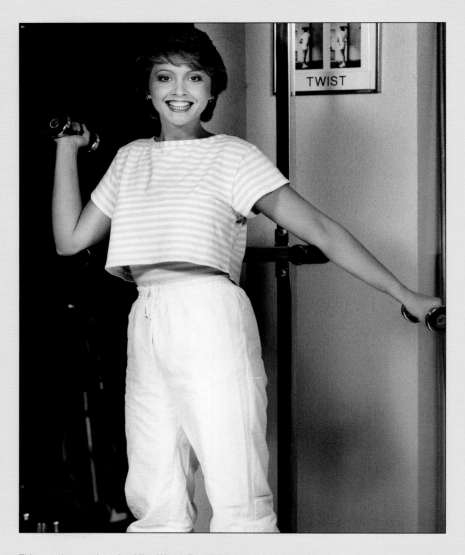

This was the morning after Miss World. To tell the truth, I hadn't much enjoyed the Miss World experience – it was everything I had often suspected it might be: a cattle market on and off stage! But the morning after, the press wanted a shot of me looking exhausted, so I put on a happy face. Then we all went out for a celebratory meal, and I was never a size eight again in my life!

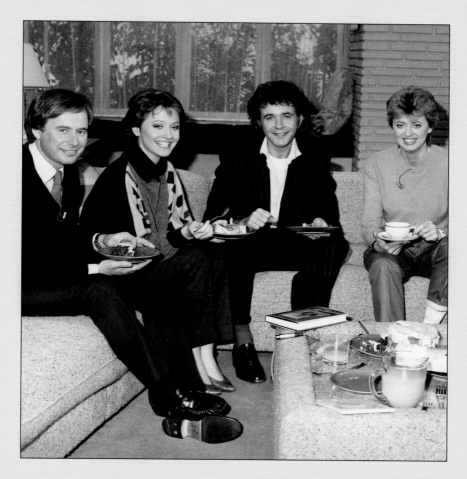

Eating was always a big part of the *TV-am* routine – especially since we had so many great resident chefs on the programme. We would all sit down on the famous sofa after the programme (often with celebrity guests like David Essex here) and munch our way through the props! I look now at pictures of myself in those days – and I can see how tiny I was. But I never thought so at the time. I was always envious of Wincey the weathergirl's lean shape!

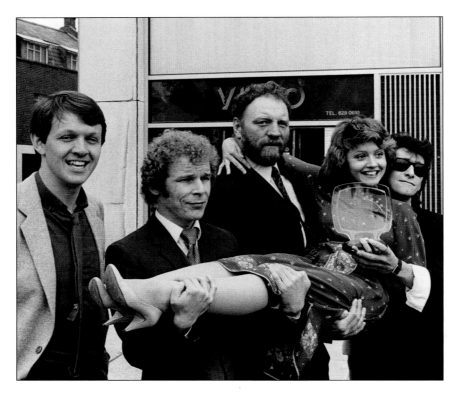

Here's a rare leggy shot of me! I think I was actually presenting an award to the cast of *Auf Wiedersehn Pet* – the photographers wanted a gimmicky pose, so we obliged. Even back then, I hated my legs so I usually covered them up in trousers. They haven't seen daylight in years!

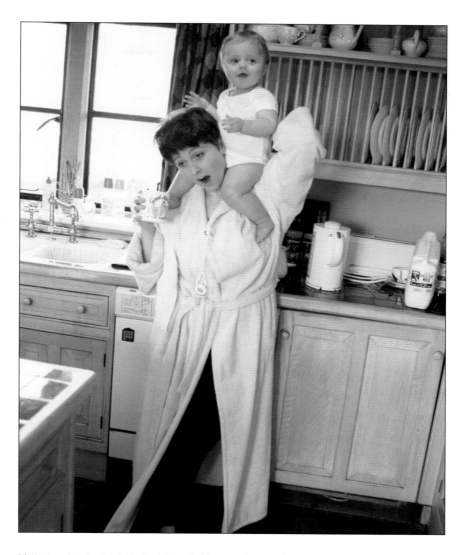

Motherhood is absolutely the best thing that has ever happened to me – but as you can see I have always specialised in big, baggy dressing gowns; not just on *Big Brother*! There's no doubt that having five children has had a major effect on my waistline – and I have certainly found it much harder to keep my weight under control as I have got older, too. This is Jake, my fourth son.

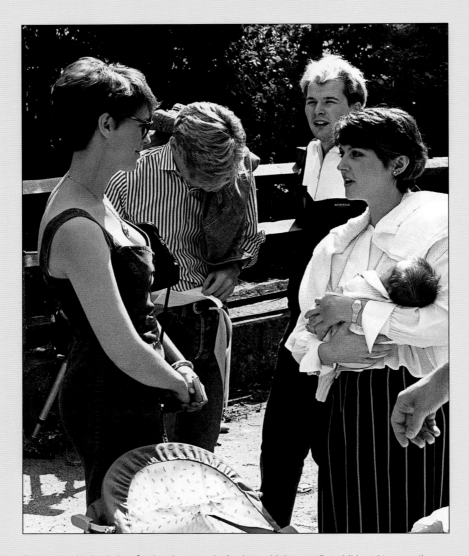

This is me with Jamie Lee Curtis — just a week after I gave birth to my first child, and two months after she had her baby. We were on the set of *A Fish Called Wanda*, back when I was reporting for *Entertainment Tonight*. I asked her how she got her figure back so quickly. She said it was simple — "I adopted"!

bedroom to get changed and was hunting for the car keys, I found one of them by the front door, changed into a tracksuit, and ready to come with me. Since then, I often find myself going along with one, or both of them. They don't stick to my side – and they don't exercise all the time I'm there. I wouldn't want them to. (I think they've discovered that there is a good social life to be had, downstairs in the coffee bar!) But it does now mean that 'going to the gym' is part of their everyday life – and that, I am sure, is important.

Tennis is an activity which really does bring us all together. Now that my smallest son can master a racquet pretty well, we can all have a good doubles game, with the odd one out as the umpire.

When you're a mum, you tend to be a role model for the rest of your family. If you are unfit and lazy, and spend most of your time watching TV, then you can only expect your family to do the same.

So try getting the whole family into your new healthy lifestyle. It's not always easy to motivate kids (and even husbands) nowadays, especially since so much of our recreation is passive – with the advent of computers and games consoles. But if you can get everyone moving, it will benefit the health of the entire family.

Here are just a few ideas which might help you get them up and at it.

Try a weekend trip to a local beauty spot, maybe for a picnic. Once you're outdoors, it'll be easier to get them playing touch football or tennis – something they'd never normally do at home.

Get a dog (or you can always offer to take your neighbour/friend's dog for a run if you don't have one). And no, I don't mean that flippantly, though clearly this is only an option if you love dogs. My neighbours recently bought a very boisterous Golden Retriever puppy. They loved animals anyway, but they deliberately got a dog because the husband had recently had a heart attack, and was told by his doctor to get walking and lose weight. My neighbour knew that having a dog would force her and her husband to exercise it. That pup has changed their entire lifestyle. I have never seen them out and about walking so much!

If you have a young child, get one of those super jogging push-chairs, specially sprung to withstand bumps at high speed. Or get a baby buggy for your bike. Another friend of mine lost all her pregnancy weight by cycling around town, with the baby in the back.

Are you tired of sitting on the sidelines? Rather than just watching your sons and daughters play football, netball, rugby and hockey, why not take a brisk walk around the games field or park? If you encourage other mums and dads to go with you, you'll promote parental camaraderie and maintain a presence at the field.

Once a week, try to get to the park or beach, or adventure playground. Attempt to coincide your visit with other families you know, so that you can all get involved with team activities. We have recently teamed up with several other families to go swimming. All it takes is a couple of phone calls – but if we can make sure we're all at the pool at the same time, we all have much more fun than if we're there alone.

chapter 7

loving yourself more than loving food

There's another reason that so many women like me have a problem with their weight – and frankly, it's not as simple nor as tangible as an ignorance of nutrition, a penchant for midnight binges or a loathing of exercise.

It's all about self-esteem. Whilst we are overloaded in the all-too-obvious spare tyre department, we are undernourished in the invisible self-esteem section. We don't have enough of it, and it's a major problem that will always be a block to losing weight successfully – and keeping it off – unless it is tackled now, head-on. Please don't snort at this point and point out that I am a TV person, so I cannot possibly have a self-esteem problem. Believe me, *if Princess Diana can suffer from low self-esteem, then anyone can*. Outwardly, many women seem confident and happy, but inwardly, they are lost.

A woman can lose her self-esteem overnight because of a major trauma or loss which devastates her life. But with many, it is a gradual process which grinds down the self-esteem over a long time. Maybe it is a boring job, a cruel or over-critical partner, a string of disastrous love affairs, a loveless existence, loneliness, or even an impossibly demanding and busy routine – self-esteem can be gradually worn down to nothing. And the sinister fact is that it can disappear without you even realising it.

I remember when a friend put it to me that I had low self-esteem, I went into immediate denial. Me? I have always been confident. Oh yes, I am confident when I absolutely need to be. Stick me in a TV studio, clip a microphone to my lapel and ask me to interview someone, or speak for twenty minutes, and I can do it, with a broad smile on my face and a twinkle in my eyes. But how many times after such a performance have I made my excuses and left while the rest of the studio crew drink the night away? Always! I want to curl up and die at most cocktail parties, and one of my biggest nightmares is walking alone into a crowded room full of partying guests.

Maybe I am just shy? Well, that may be so. But half the time I refuse such invitations because I feel awkward, or I don't think I look the way I should, or I think that no one will really care whether I am there or not, so I might as well be at home. That isn't shyness, that's low self-esteem! Mind you, it doesn't help when you know a press photographer is following you around, lurking in the shadows, just so they can get a picture of your bum. I distinctly remember spending a whole week trying to dodge a *Today* newspaperman who was compiling a photo report on Britain's biggest bums. I had to wear a winter coat all week. It was July!

Loss of self-esteem, while difficult for the sufferer to detect, can have easy-to-detect signs for everyone else. They usually show in a woman's appearance. Has she put on a lot of weight? Has she bothered to have her hair cut or coloured recently? Does she wear make-up to go out – even to the shops? Has she lost her sense of fashion? When she goes out clothes shopping, does she ever buy anything for herself – or does she always come back with something for the children?

I have interviewed women who say that they've lost a sense of who they really are, and that they often feel invisible at home to their husbands or children – a bit like one of those Under House Parlour Maids in Victorian times, who were always slaving away at domestic chores, but whose presence was not acknowledged at all by the Mistress or Master of the home! Of course, if that's happened to you – then you have only yourself to blame. If *you* hadn't let it happen, if you had delegated some of those horrible domestic chores, if you hadn't always given up your place on the sofa, at the table or even in charge of the remote control, then they would have sat up and taken some notice of you. The point is, though, that it happened gradually – and each chipping away of the way you are valued in the home, takes away more of your self-value. It becomes a downward spiral, and is very difficult to reverse.

It happens a lot to women when they have children, because maternal instincts programme you to sacrifice everything for your children. Of course, what Nature intended was for you to sacrifice everything necessary for your child's health and safety. Many women are able to keep a very sensible perspective on that. They think of themselves, and their partners too. But often, women find themselves so unbearably busy – so stretched – that they lose sight of the fact that *they* matter, too. I call it 'Leggings at the School Gate' syndrome. You can tell them a mile off. They're the women who are gathered at the school exit, waiting for their children at the end of the day, and they're dressed in a uniform baggy T-shirt or anorak, and shapeless leggings. If you asked them why they wore that 'uniform', they would say it is comfortable and practical, and easily washed!

At the other end of the spectrum are the Tennis Princesses (and I have seen many of these, too, at school gates!) who pull up in their hatchbacks, spreadeagle their cars over two car parking spaces, and block everyone else's exit. They're still wearing their tennis dresses or golf shorts from an afternoon with the girlfriends, and their stick-thin wrists are almost breaking under the weight of Rolexes and charm bracelets. Oh yes, and their little Tristrams and Britneys are the terrors of the fifth form!

It has always been my ambition to be one of them, or at least to look so impossibly relaxed and carefree, with the body, car, and bank balance to match! I am just not built that way, in more ways than one.

At home, I have to constantly remind myself that I must delegate jobs – to other adults and to the children – rather than sigh and get on with doing them myself. If I am not careful, I find myself laying the table, taking the bins out, clearing up the mess, mowing the lawn – and all because it is easier to do it myself than go and peel my four strapping sons off their computer screens, explain to them how I want it done, argue with them, remind them and then check up on them afterwards – just to make sure it was done!

If you even find yourself thinking like that – or if you are already better at it than I am – then stop it at once! You are creating a huge problem for yourself, and it will grow even bigger!

Get a grip! Examine your own view of yourself. How do you rate your own value, on a scale of one to ten?

It is never too late to re-take charge of your life – or even change it fundamentally.

Those around you may react a little defensively – after all, you are changing their lives too, by refusing to be a doormat. They may pooh-pooh your efforts to change. They may say supposedly comforting things like: 'you are lovely just the way you are!' They may scoff at your ambitions, laugh at your efforts to diet, patronise you or mock your ideas of going back to college, getting a job, improving yourself. Don't let it get to you. They're just jealous, or scared, or feel threatened by the thought of you changing into someone they cannot handle. People are often frightened of change.

But it doesn't have to threaten any of the people or things you value. Finding a new lifestyle will not alter the person you are inside. It won't make you a selfish person – just a self-aware one. And it will make you happier.

So how do you improve your self-esteem?

Well, one way would be to go into therapy, find out when and where your esteem took a downwards spin, go back to your childhood, analyse what lessons and habits you may have learned from your mother or father. However, if you are a pretty regular woman, with a weight problem and enough determination to do something about it (and, since you are reading this book, I guess you are!) then you may be able to fix things yourself, without too much introspection. However you go about it, you will ultimately be faced with this question:

What can I do from now on to turn myself into a more confident, mature and content person – someone who has high self-esteem and a happier life because of it?

You have got to learn to love yourself.

Sounds very strange. In fact, it sounds selfish and self-centred and all those things we were taught NOT to be by our mothers.

It sounds like psycho-babble.

It sounds impossible!

But you can learn how to do it – and you will find it worthwhile, I promise.

I remember, on *Good Morning with Anne and Nick*, we featured a group of viewers who wanted to lose weight. They were all hugely puzzled as to why they had put on so much weight in the first place, and then utterly confounded when they had tried everything they could to slim, and failed. We brought them into the studio, where they were advised by various different weight loss counsellors and fitness experts. One lady was required to look at herself in the mirror, and she was asked which parts of her body did she approve of? Her eyes began to well up with tears, as she struggled to find something nice to say about just one part. In the end, after more tears, she conceded that her ear lobes were OK.

Her *ear lobes*.

It was so sad. Having only just met her, I could see a lovely lady, with a pleasing face and a happy, chatty manner. She could see nothing about herself which she liked at all. It taught me a lesson I will never forget. That in this hurly-burly, frantically busy world, where we are often expected to be 'superwomen' in our jobs, in our daily domestic lives, in bed, in the kitchen – the single one person we forget to look after well is so often *ourselves*.

But hey – let's stop all the criticism! At least you have got yourself this far! You want to change, and you want to lose weight, look gorgeous, feel slim, be fit... Well, your mental attitude is crucial.

We have already seen how so many of us have an emotional relationship with food – how we eat to comfort ourselves, or use food as a reward for good behaviour. Now you have to learn to think like someone who is going to succeed, like someone who deserves to do well, feel trim and fit and skinny, like a champion. You have got to practise visualisation. You must be able to close your eyes and see yourself as slim. It's got to be such a potent and powerful image that it pops into your brain and reminds you of what you are going to become.

It seems paradoxical, but you cannot think yourself slim unless you start learning to love your body now – *even before* it is slim and lithe and fit.

After all, how can you do the best for your body if you hate it?

How can you pamper it, soften it in relaxing bath oils, cosset it with the creamiest moisturisers, scent it with the sexiest perfumes, how can you even take it along to the gym or to the park and give it a good workout if you loathe your body?

You have got to learn to love your body and you have got to start doing that *now*, if you want it to be appealing, stay gorgeous and become even more attractive over the next few months. Start loving yourself – you really are worth it. You *have* to value yourself in order to take the next steps: to eat the foods which are going to take the most care of your body, and exercise in order to get it looking its best. You have to value something to invest in it, don't you?

Think of it like the little car you always wanted, or maybe like the first car you ever had. It wasn't the most expensive model available, it wasn't even the latest, factory-fresh example – but it was yours. It may even have had its cranky moments: mine (a little, white, old and battered MG Midget) leaked in bad weather, and burned more oil than petrol – but it carried me around the country, visiting friends and family and taking me on exciting romantic trips, and I loved it. It was a little gem, even though it wasn't like those on the front cover of the car magazines. I bought it the best oil I could afford. I polished and waxed it. I even nagged my Dad to overhaul the engine, because he knew about such things! I really took care of it, even though it was a little rusty and very temperamental.

What you have got to do is think of your body in the same way. It may not be magazine-perfect. It may not be just like Cindy Crawford's. It might even leak occasionally – or need the odd jump-start on a cold day, but it is yours, and it needs love and care. I had to learn this lesson too, when I came out of the *Big Brother* house. In the newspapers, all the headlines said horrid things about my body. Words like 'gargantuan', 'massive' and 'beached whale' stung like a thousand wasps, but I had to learn to see myself differently in the mirror. As big as I was, I started to appreciate little bits of me. I stood in front of the mirror, too. First of all, I quite liked most of my face – that was the easiest bit. Next, I found that I liked my feet – they have always been quite small and dainty. Next, I found that I was still quite proud of my cleavage, and could still find clothes that showed it to its best advantage – it was even quite sexy, so some admirers said.

And so I worked on it, learning to love myself a little bit more every day. Frankly, this was something I had never, ever done – not even in my slimmest days. I had never liked my body, and so had never treated it particularly well. While friends got excited about new face creams and body lotions, I couldn't see the point. This time, I vowed to take more care of my legs! Somewhere in the back of a cupboard, I found a lovely body lotion and I applied it every day, before bed. Within weeks, the skin on my legs and the backs of my arms was smoother. With every week, I was able to count the positive steps forward – smoother skin, a pound or two lost, a slightly flatter tummy. Cindy Crawford might have died rather than wake up in my body, but I was beginning to feel more pleased about it!

Ten steps to loving yourself

1. Take off all your clothes and look at yourself in a full-length mirror

Wow! That takes some courage. Now list three parts of your body that you really like. If three don't come to mind – *work at it* until you find three parts that you can eventually be positive about. Your toes, your ears? Your eyes? Do this every day – and then, every week, gradually increase the amount of parts to four things, then five, and so on. It's a difficult exercise, but a very useful one, so take it fairly seriously, please! Apparently, the part of the body always rated highest by women is the face – even though we all admit we're not cover girls. That's because we are more accepting of our faces, because we are so used to them. So, three or four times a week, spend a few minutes perusing your naked body in a mirror. Gradually you will teach yourself that you can find a positive approach.

2. Stop asking for others' approval

Are you always asking for reassurance from friends, your partner or even your kids? Are you the one who asks: 'Does my bum look big in this?' Well, stop! Make up your own mind whether or not you look good in something. And try to be positive, remember! Don't constantly weigh yourself, check yourself out in every mirror, and compulsively compare yourself to every other woman in the room. If you cannot give up this need for reassurance straight away, cut down your requests for it. For instance, if you're going to a party, make a deal with yourself that you'll ask your husband only once if you look fat.

3. Be sensual with yourself

Take a long, hot bath in relaxing aromatherapy oils. Slowly drink something very cold on a hot day; put a soothing lotion all over your body; soak your tootsies in warm water or a foot spa if you have one, in front of the TV; go swimming in the sea, a river or lake; get a sauna or a massage; spend an afternoon listening to your favourite music or watch a sensuous movie; get a little tattoo (a fake one works just as well!) in a naughty place. Indulge just for the sake of indulgence – just try not to make it food! Do something that gives you physical pleasure every day.

4. Stop complaining about yourself

Don't moan to others about your little imperfections! Women love to sit together pulling themselves to bits, but it would do us all more good if we got together and praised each other's abilities and looks. Try opting for other positive experiences – maybe go for a leisurely walk in the park with a friend, and gossip while you enjoy feeding the ducks.

5. See your body as the passport to a new you

It's not the barrier to a new life – it is the way forward. It is so ironic that hating oneself for being overweight can be one reason you stay that way. That's why nurturing yourself is so important – or you will never end the cycle of self-defeat.

You need to work on being your own best friend instead of your own worst enemy. And remember, you may feel right now that you'd like a body transplant, but ask your body and it probably feels all it needs is a *brain* transplant – and your body would look like a million dollars in just a few months.

6. Visualise

Practise visualisation techniques. Close your eyes and see yourself as a slim person, wearing a particular outfit. Now imagine it so fiercely that you can actually feel you are that superslim, sexy you. Taste it, smell it! Feel those lovely clothes on your body. Feel how good it is to move freely, without clothes being tight and awkward, without all that extra weight to carry around. Do this at least once a day.

7. Treat your body as a temple!

It's odd, but so many women don't really care what food and drink they put in their own body, but they worry about every little morsel that goes into their children! I have heard mums say 'I won't let the little one drink cola – it's so unhealthy…' and yet they are pouring the stuff down their own throats. This goes for all sorts of things from sweets to fatty foods. Just because we are adults doesn't mean we don't deserve tender, loving care! Similarly, look after your skin, your hair, your nails – your overall health. Get a medical checkup, book into a Well Woman clinic and ensure that everything inside is OK. You are a precious commodity (just think how difficult and expensive it would be to replace you!) so take care!

8. Make some 'me' time

I used to be one of those people who said I would like to make 'me' time, but I simply didn't have the time. My day was too crammed to allow anything else in. Then a friend pointed out: 'If one of your children was ill, and needed daily physiotherapy – you would make the time, wouldn't you?' Of course you would – somehow. The truth is, if we consider something important enough, we can find the time, even if it is very hard. So push yourself up the priority list and give yourself thirty minutes a day to relax and read a magazine, sit and think, soak your feet, or just meditate. Or find a new hobby. I have just taken up painting and find it wonderfully relaxing and absorbing.

9. Try an alternative therapy

Some people swear by these 'alternative' therapies – well, why not try one and see what it does for you? I had a go at reflexology to cure my hayfever (I didn't stick at it long enough to know), aromatherapy to help me get a better night's sleep (brilliant) and just a few months ago, I tried hypnotherapy with a hypnotist who specialised in weight loss. Rather than 'going under' and being mesmerised, I thought it was more like sessions of re-affirmation of all the sensible advice I had learned, and reminders of what I wanted – like visualisation. I was very impressed. At any rate, it was a positive and imaginative thing to be doing for *me*. Whatever therapy you try, remember that it doesn't have to be expensive to be good: my library stocks great meditation videos which I've found really helpful.

10. Give yourself and your things a makeover

Get a new haircut or go a new colour, have a girly night where you can do each other's hair, nails, make-up or mini-facials! What about one new outfit, or some wardrobe swapping with your best friend? Revive your make-up bag, go to the beauty counter and ask for help with some new colours (don't forget to ask for some free samples, and that way you won't need to spend any money, but can still end up with a free makeover!). Next: makeover your bedroom, or at least one room or corner of the house that you see as 'yours'. That's one good thing about being divorced! I made my bedroom over completely – everything is cream-coloured, with a variety of textures like silk, fur and linen. I bought some lush, showpiece plants (and have even managed to keep them alive!) and a pair of large, Venetian-style mirrors. It is now a bedroom where I could happily take Mr Right, should he ever come calling. And another good thing about cream bedcovers – you daren't eat anywhere near them! Tidying up and binning old newspapers, old clothes etc also works wonders for your morale: you'll feel a sense of achievement, plus you'll have worked off a few calories in the meantime!

chapter 8

how I got on

I think the meal I miss most is elevenses. A cup of coffee and a good dunking biscuit was something worth looking forward to in the morning. I miss the satisfaction I used to feel from sitting down and just savouring them.

I know that I am free to have them if I want – and I have tried. But they just don't taste the same any more – and that's almost the saddest part!

Coffee, tea, even my old tipple, Bacardi and cola – none of them taste the same any more. They're OK, but somehow they're no longer delicious. Maybe they never were. Maybe they were just a habit.

Have you ever heard children exclaim: 'ugh!' when they try a small taste of beer, or wine? Then they ask: 'Why do you like it, Mummy?' and you find yourself explaining that it is an 'acquired taste'.

People say that about cigarettes, too, don't they? Everyone hates their first ever drag – it makes them choke, cough and spit. They have to work at it, in order to develop a taste. Daft, isn't it?

I sometimes wonder if a lot of our tastes are only desirable to us because we have acquired them over a lifetime – tastes like sugar.

I was brought up in a home where everyone took sugar in their tea.

I had a wonderful Great Aunt Lil, who used to stay with us from time to time. She was crippled with arthritis, and used to hobble around with a zimmer frame, but she was a great mate of mine.

One of the skills she took great pleasure in teaching me was how to make a pot of tea.

When I look back, I realise it was a very canny, sneaky thing to do. Because from then on, if anyone in the house ever fancied a cuppa, it would be little Anne who would get up and make it.

'Ooh! Anne can really make a brilliant cup of tea,' they would all sigh. Hmm.

However, as I was saying, we all took one or two teaspoonsful of sugar each in our tea.

Only when I became a body-conscious teenager, did I think about giving up sugar.

I remember I went cold turkey on it. I just gave up one day, and kept going through sheer willpower. I thought that I might allow myself to have sugar in my tea occasionally as a treat.

One day, I realised that I was enjoying tea without sugar. When I tried sugar in my tea, it tasted absolutely revolting. Not just sweet, but almost a chemical taste!

I am sure you have experienced something like this, too. It makes you wonder, doesn't it, what we could quite happily live without if we were forced to, or if we chose to?

I changed over to healthy eating as soon as I had finished Jason's book, and then met him and discussed the finer points of juicing. At first, it wasn't difficult at all – I just made a mental check on all the foods I would normally have eaten, and asked myself what it was made from – what was in them, what had been added and taken away.

Then, I mentally chucked them in the trash can.

Some of it just required a change of approach during shopping. For instance, if I was in the supermarket buying bread (or flour to make bread), I just ensured that it had the word wholemeal on it. When I first came home with wholemeal pittas instead of the bright, white ones, the children rebelled. But they're over it now – once I explained why the difference was important.

Fruit and vegetable shopping was pretty straightforward. I tried to buy organic whenever I could, for the items I was going to eat raw – like avocados, carrots, cucumbers and tomatoes, and most fruits. Other vegetables, such as potatoes, onions, leeks, peppers, sweetcorn, I am not so fussy about whether they're organic or not. Many experts say that, by the time you've peeled and cooked them, there's barely a difference, so that is where I economise a little.

I did notice a huge saving when I came to the bottled drinks department – because I decided to boycott the lot. I did, however, buy orange and apple juice as before, because the children love them.

But I should take out shares in tuna. I don't think I have ever eaten so much! Salmon, too!

I have a friend, Dave, who does a very physical job – a tremendously fit guy, but someone who was several stones overweight last year. Then he went on a diet he invented himself – the tuna roll diet. Whenever he felt hungry, he just demolished a roll, jam-packed with tuna and salad. He lost count of how many he ate – but that was all he had during the day, when before, he would have snacked on chocolate and crisps. Well, the weight just fell off him, over the summer. He is now lithe and lean. And if I say any more, he'll blush. So I bow to Dave and the power of tuna – and include it in my food plan nearly every day. It is so handy, protein-packed and easy to prepare. Become a tunatarian! (Dolphin friendly, of course!)

I should also invest in a salad leaves farm, oh, and a Balsamic vinegar plant – I have become so addicted to salads, drizzled with that lovely dressing. Again, if you buy your salad leaves in a prepared packet, it makes meal preparation so easy, but they can be expensive so what I tend to do is bulk wash a load of vegetable leaves, pat them dry and store them in the vegetable drawer in the fridge!

There's no doubt, I spent my first weeks having to seriously think before I ate every meal. If the rest of the family were sitting down to a Sunday roast – what could I eat?

Well, actually, it was quite easy. The chicken is healthy (although I avoid it because I am vegetarian), so were all the veggies. I would, however, avoid the Yorkshire pudding (because I haven't even attempted to make it with wholemeal flour yet) and the stuffing (refined wheatflours and lots of processed ingredients).

Foods which are a mass of different ingredients, or those where you cannot even tell what they're made of, are 'mystery foods'. You often see mystery foods at parties – strangely coloured mush wrapped inside deep fried pastry wedges, or blobs of something creamy on a cracker. Mystery foods should be avoided at all costs because you can't tell if they're made entirely of healthy ingredients.

Of course, it sounds and feels strange to dismiss some foods as 'unhealthy' when the rest of the family are eating them. The truth is though, my concentration on buying and eating healthier foods has rubbed off on most of the meals I now cook for everyone. It's just that I am extra picky, because I am the one trying to lose weight.

The early morning buzz and whir of the juicer and blender in my kitchen has had an interesting effect though – on my sons, who don't usually take any interest in such gadgets. Suddenly we have banana smoothies, mango milkshakes and fresh orange and pineapple juices on the breakfast table. I am very proud of that! My 14 year old son, Jamie, can prepare a wonderful avocado and prawn starter, and my youngest, Conor, makes a fine home-made orange juice ice lolly.

Healthy habits are catching – and that's exciting.

It has been the same with exercise, too. Since I started the trampolining, everyone suddenly wants to get on it. (And they're better at it than me, too, which is very annoying!)

I cannot say I absolutely enjoyed the first few weeks of going to the gym. It honestly was a drag – because it was such hard work! Even the easiest of workouts on the treadmill (ten minutes) or the cross-trainer (five minutes and I was a wreck) made me feel pretty disheartened.

I booked myself a personal trainer – just so that I wouldn't give up and go home – and I can honestly confess that if it hadn't been for the feeling that I would let him down, I would have backed away from the gym and convinced myself that I could do as well at home.

But Chris, my trainer, was incredibly patient – and so I stuck at it. Gradually, very gradually, I found I could do more without wanting to curl up and die. I managed one day to do a full ten minutes on that blessed cross-trainer, and felt like I had won the Olympics.

Funny, too, that one of the most off-putting aspects of going along to a gym for the first time is the idea that you are the only one there who's overweight, unfit and sweating like a dockyard navvy. After a while, you realise that at least half the clientele look like you. A quarter are actually fatter than you – and yes, there is always the other 25% of beautiful, slim young men and women, elegantly sporting the sleekest of lycra outfits. You learn not to hate them, just envy their outfits and swear to yourself that you'll get into one of those little black numbers one day!

So there I was, reading all my food labels, questioning myself before every mouthful, and working my socks off in the gym.

I was feeling healthier. Gone was the feeling of lethargy in the morning. Maybe I didn't quite leap out of bed – but I certainly felt human. No headaches, or muzzy-head.

I was feeling fitter. I could run after the children without getting breathless. I could go up and downstairs without panting.

One day, I was filming with an ITN crew at a London hospital. We were there to make a report about cot death, and were interviewing some new mums on the maternity ward. Waiting for ages, with all our equipment, at the ground floor lift doors, we realised the lift was never going to come. Instead we would have to walk up the six flights of stairs.

Weeks before, I would have dreaded the thought. By the time I got to the top, all puffed and pink, I would have felt hot and sticky, and far too uncomfortable to happily film a piece to camera.

On this day, though, I climbed the stairs without flinching. It was such a tiny achievement – and entirely unknown and invisible to anyone with me. But it felt so good! That's when I knew I would return to that wretched cross-trainer the next day. It had given me back my leg muscles!

So things were looking good, after just a couple of months of free and easy healthy eating. Except that things were not looking so good on the scales. Yes, I had lost six pounds. That sort of weight loss would please any slimming counsellor nowadays. After all, they all think that slow weight loss is best. But it seemed painfully slow to me.

So when I started the 21 Day Kickstart plan I never, in my wildest dreams, thought I would ever salivate at the mere thought of an avocado salad. I would have laughed if you'd told me that I would manage to get through the day on a couple of pints of apple, celery, cucumber and avocado smoothie. But I did it – because I had already got myself into a mode of thinking that was telling me: 'get healthy, get happy'.

I think if you embarked on the 21 day plan straight away, without getting used to the healthy eating ideas, you would find it very restrictive, very hard-going. But once those new ideas are firmly in your psyche, it's really not that difficult.

For those first few days, when I was only drinking juices, I just kept myself as busy as possible, especially in the evenings. And I went to bed early, treating the whole experience a bit like a long weekend at a health farm.

By day four, I was really feeling hungry – but excited, too, as the scales were starting to move, quite dramatically!

I lost 13 pounds in the first 13 days – magic! A week later, my 21 days were up and I had lost one stone and two pounds. I was so relieved! It was like a huge weight had been lifted from my shoulders (except that it was from all over my body!).

I think I had begun to convince myself that I would never be slim again. Now I knew I would.

chapter 9

Pitfalls! A: hitting a plateau

Dear Diary:

Monday May 12

If I eat any more tuna I will start looking like a fish. I am so fed up. Been eating nothing but fruit and tuna, tuna and fruit for days – and I haven't lost a pound. Rang Jason. He says just keep going, but I am beginning to think I've had enough. Gave in and had a Bacardi and coke tonight. What a way to start the week. Now I feel a total failure.

Tuesday May 13

Woke up tired, with a slightly sick feeling – and a headache. I feel like it's 'the morning after the night before', but I only had *one* drink last night! Had a huge breakfast to get rid of the sick feeling, and then felt worse. Had a big lunch too – a big stir-fry and two baked potatoes. Jason rang and I dared not tell him about the drink – nor the potatoes. He has banned me from weighing myself so often – he says I should only get on the scales once a fortnight. Am going to bed with a large glass of *water*. Very exciting. I wouldn't mind all this if I were only losing weight. I am starving hungry and yet I can't lose a pound. It doesn't make any sense.

Wednesday May 14

Saw Chris the trainer at the gym and told him my woes. He thinks I'm not eating enough. Gave me a really tough workout – absolutely exhausted. Am eating healthily again, today. Feel better. Went back to the gym this evening and did another hour on my own. Surely things should move now?

Thursday May 15

Weighed myself again. I've actually *put on* two pounds. How the hell? Interviewed today for *It Shouldn't Happen To A TV Presenter!* and had to be very jolly, but I really feel like jumping off a tall building. What the hell is going on? I rang Jason. He says I shouldn't weigh myself all the time – and he said just keep going.

Friday May 16

Weighed myself again. I have lost two pounds. That's better – but it still only puts me back where I was on Monday – and already a week has gone by! Drove to Droitwich to open a new community centre for mums and babies. Had a nightmare time avoiding all the food and nibbles being offered! But I stuck to my guns – came home and ate two tuna salads.

Saturday May 17

No change in my weight at all. Took the kids out to Pizza Hut for lunch. Managed to stick to a Caesar salad while they all had garlic bread and pizza. Very proud of myself. Nearly tempted to have a Bacardi tonight – so instead, I poured the lot down the sink. Feel very holy.

Sunday May 18

I haven't weighed myself today at all – instead I woke up early and did my exercises and listened to my retuning CD. Friends over for lunch (Katie and kids) – I cooked a huge roast. Tuna salad for me! Katie brought me a bottle of Bacardi to say thank you!

Monday May 19

Had my picture taken for the *Daily Mail* column – I think I still look very fat. Went to the gym and did a big workout. Still haven't gone near the scales – I just plodded on with the healthy eating programme. Took the kids swimming tonight, still hate myself in swimming costume. Will I ever wear a bikini again in my life?

Tuesday May 20

Man called Kevin came to the house today to show me his new 'PowerPlates' exercise machine – the latest gizmo from the States. It's a huge vibrating plate, which you do your exercises on – and it makes each exercise ten times more powerful, so you don't have to exercise for very long. It feels really strange but if it helps… I'll do anything! Kevin's going to install one at the gym so I can work on it there. A good food day, though I was a bit tempted by the Bacardi tonight. A + P came around for a drink – and I had a Bacardi, dammit!

Wednesday May 21

Been invited to a *I'm A Celebrity Get Me Out Of Here!* do tonight – and also on to *Richard and Judy* to judge their art competition. Couldn't do both – so plumped for R+J. Richard was very kind – said he thought I'd lost a lot of weight! (Bet he says that to all the girls.) But isn't it amazing how a little compliment can make you feel good? Too busy to go to the gym today – am worried now that I am letting things slip. Weighed myself tonight. I've put on four pounds. I am going to go mad.

Thursday May 22

Weighed myself again. I have lost four pounds – but still that lands me back in square one! I am so fed up, I just cannot believe it. I am eating so much less than I usually do – I just couldn't eat any less than this or I would faint. What can I do? Went to the gym again, but felt so tired I came home again after just five minutes. Poured the entire contents of Bacardi bottle down the sink – in case I get tempted. I know it's a waste of money, but I don't care now. Made a huge Jason-type juice and had nothing else all day.

Friday May 23

Been busy all day working at the TV studios. Came home at 6 and J came with me to the gym. We had a really good time, competing against each other. Then had dinner – pan fried salmon and veggies with large bottle of AquaLibra (dangerous living!). J thinks maybe I haven't lost pounds on the scales because I am developing muscle. He says my body looks a little slimmer. Maybe I am doing too much exercise?

Saturday May 24

Busy all day at school: 'Founder's Day'. Mrs B had made 'Coronation Quorn' especially for me – and it was very tasty. Saved from eating the lot by the rain – which bucketed down all afternoon. Went to the gym again, just for twenty minutes, and then joined the kids for a swim. The trouble with swimming is – it makes me so hungry. Had a long bath instead and went to bed early.

Sunday May 25

Had a thousand little boys round for birthday party. Surprised to find I was not tempted by all the sausages on sticks and peanut butter sarnies. In

pitfalls! a: hitting a plateau

fact, I never want to see one again. What did I have? A tuna salad! By the time I had everyone in bed, I was so exhausted, I gave in to a bowl of Rice Krispies. Now I am worried I have blown the healthy eating plan again – but if just one bowl of cereal blows me off course, then life isn't worth living. I am dying to weigh myself again, and if I haven't lost any weight now, I really will die.

Monday May 26

Got on the scales – and guess what? I have lost two measly pounds. I really feel like giving up – except that everyone says 'just keep going – in the end, you will lose weight' and I am just clinging to that. But it's very hard…

Just looking at my diary from last year, and reading the words tapped into my laptop last thing at night, I can still sense the feelings of despair.

After the initial euphoria of the first few weeks on Jason's 21 Day Kickstart plan when the weight seemed to drip off me, suddenly I hit a horrible plateau – and that's how things progressed for quite a few weeks. I swear even Jason's resolve was beginning to waver – and those around me must have concluded that I must be secretly stashing food away in my bedroom and going back to my old ways of midnight munching!

But I wasn't. I really was trying hard to keep all my eating healthy – and pretty restricted. I had re-introduced carbohydrates to my daytime eating, but I was still cutting out all carbs after six (which I think is a pretty good habit anyway), apart from, of course, when I gave in to a little drinkie.

It's interesting, now, to see that I never gave a thought to how big that little drinkie was. In truth, the amounts of spirits we serve at home from our

121

own drinks cabinets are probably twice or three times the size of a pub measure.

But even that – and the odd bowl of cornflakes (and of course, any diet should be able to absorb that once in a while) – couldn't explain the awful stalemate I'd reached.

That's the trouble with plateaux – there's just no explaining them. And you are bound to hit one. If you already have, please don't despair. They are a pain, but there are things you can do.

There are a lot of pseudo-scientific theories as to why people hit plateaux. And you can tie yourself up in knots trying to understand whether your metabolic rate equals this, whether you're building muscle or you're burning fat. But plateaux generally happen because of one of two reasons:

1. Either you have become lazy or absent-minded about your new health regime – but you don't realise you're letting things slack.
2. Or – your body has got used to what you're doing and you need to rev up the engine a little more.

To be brutally frank, the first reason is the most common reason for plateaux. You think you are being strict, but you're not. Now I look back, I think that may have been what happened to me.

Only one thing for it – start keeping a food diary. Make a note of everything going in, and you'll probably see where things are going wrong. The odd snack here and there that you thought wouldn't count, the little evening drinkie (that's really a triple shot!) with those nibbles. The subconscious belief that you're doing quite well and you deserve a little hidden 'treat'… That's why things aren't moving.

By jotting down everything that passes your lips, you'll be able to see whether you've inadvertently settled into some counterproductive eating habits. (One woman I talked to at the gym told me she'd been shocked to find that a few too many boiled sweets and 'healthy' energy bars had sneaked into her diet when she wasn't looking.) And by logging how often and how long you work out, you'll be able to validate your exercise regime. Through these 'reality checks', you may discover that the diet you thought you were sticking to so well is really not quite as moderate as you'd thought, or that your four workouts a week is really only two. (I think that happened to me, as well!)

But if you still find you really have hit a plateau, and you really are keeping to your food ideals, then you must look at exercise.

Are you getting enough?

Our body needs energy for two reasons: (1) To tick over, and (2) To support any additional activity.

Every second of our life, our body is constantly active. For example, it takes in and transports oxygen to every cell, muscle, tissue and organ. It builds, re-builds, maintains, repairs and cleans itself. It counters infection. It maintains a constant safe temperature and regulates millions of chemical reactions. So even when we sleep or do nothing, the body is actively ticking over. About 70% of our energy is used in this ticking over process.

The moment we get up or start moving around, we need extra energy. The more active we are and the more exercise we take, the more energy we need.

But where do we get energy from?

Our body has two sources of available energy: one is food, and the other is stored energy in the form of glycogen, fat and lean tissue or muscle.

In order to lose weight we must eat less food than our body needs to convert into energy. In other words, if you are overweight, it is because your food intake is greater than your energy requirement. One remedy is to eat less.

For example:

If we need 1500 calories a day to tick over and 200 calories for additional activities, then our total energy requirement is 1700 calories. Therefore, if we take in 1600 calories from food, our body will take 100 calories worth of energy from our fat stores, and we will lose weight.

Now there's a problem: our body doesn't like to lose weight. It's not interested in being slim. It is interested only in survival. So if our food intake is insufficient, it starts to slow down in order to conserve energy and boost its chances of survival. This is why weight loss tends to slow down as we continue to diet, and why you may feel you've hit a plateau.

That's why you have to make sure you are eating enough. So – apart from when you're on the 21 Day Kickstart plan (if you choose to do it) – you should be eating well at each meal time, as long as it is all healthy, whole food. Eat too little and your metabolism will slow down. Have a look at the '10 FAQs about metabolism' section on page 252 and you'll probably be able to find something that'll help speed things up again.

But it's not just about volume of food – it's also about quality. Starving yourself denies your body the balance of vitamins and nutrients it needs. On top of that, you'll start to feel depressed and tired – two key reasons people give up.

No, you've got to exercise. And if you are already doing some, step it up – just a little. Or change your exercise routine. If you have done quite well with the exercise bike, try adding five minutes skipping afterwards. If you're quite settled doing ten or fifteen minutes on the treadmill, try a two minute run around the garden – but keep it up for a solid two minutes. Believe me, it's far harder than it sounds! If you're in the gym, ask an instructor to show you some exercises on a different set of equipment. That way you won't get too bored.

If you're working out alone, try getting into a class, where you might be inspired to work harder by the other people around you. You can also try working out to faster music than you're used to; your body will probably want to keep pace with the rhythm all on its own.

Then, too, consider incorporating into your daily life some other ways to increase your burn, like parking your car further from work and walking briskly over that distance, or taking the stairs instead of the lift. And when the phone rings, don't necessarily reach for the closest extension. (One study I read reckoned that the average person would walk an additional 17 miles a year if there was only one phone in the house!) The point is to find any way at all to raise your activity levels.

Keep focused on the bigger picture. Be proud of the fact that you've made some healthy positive changes for yourself. Your body is going through an adjustment period right now and needs some time, so don't do what I did. Don't become obsessed by the scales, instead keep thinking of the positive changes you were going to make, and see how many days of the week you can stick to those. The weight will start to shift again.

I can honestly say that I have now learned that you *can* get through plateaux – and, in a nutshell, the only way is this:

1. If your eating plan is right, then just doggedly keep on going.
2. Perk up your exercising – but don't overdo things.
3. Stay focused on your aims.

4. Keep off the scales – they sometimes tell you more than you need to know!

I hit several plateaux – but I did get through them. You can, too!

chapter 10

Pitfalls! B: falling off the wagon

(and those who can push you off it)

After one particularly awful plateau, when I hadn't lost a pound for what seemed like weeks (although, when I look back in the diary now, I find it was only about eight days!) I came up with a new idea.

I thought I'd go on a fast!

I came up with the idea when I was surfing the internet. I was actually working, researching my children's book which is set in the English Civil War. One minute, I was perusing a load of historical websites about Oliver Cromwell – and the next minute I found I'd turned to a search engine, and my fingers were automatically typing in the words 'slimming' and then 'plateau'.

Up came a host of wonderful pages, mostly suggesting dodgy-sounding drugs you could only get by mail order if you live in America. But there were also quite a few sites, many from New Age type organisations, recommending fasts of various sorts.

There were several with whole pages devoted to 'juice fasts'. Since I was already into juicing, I thought I'd read on. Maybe this was something I could do quite easily, I thought.

Basically, the idea was to drink/eat nothing but water and homemade juices – in some cases, for as long as a month. Apart from some spurious claims about allowing you to get in touch with 'your real self' and cleansing and detoxifying your body, it was also meant to be a pretty effective way of losing a lot of weight very fast.

Now, I'm not daft. But I was desperate, so I thought I would give it a try – if only for a week. Of course, it would have helped enormously if I'd been able to leave all my domestic cares behind, and jet off to a monastery in Tibet for the week. But I had things to do at home.

Ah well, I thought. At least it will cut down on all the cooking – and preparation of tuna salads!

I stuck to my favourite juice blend – apple, pineapple, cucumber, celery and avocado – and made plenty of it. My kitchen looked like Covent Garden market at sunrise. I was enthusiastic, almost excited!

Of course, I know now what I was doing… I was clinging to a new idea like a slimmer buys into a new diet. But, I thought, it's entirely healthy, if a little extreme – what harm can it do?

Two days in, and I was still fine. I didn't even feel weak. In fact, I was energised. I really do think that a morning juice is a tonic.

Days three and four, and I did start to feel rather hungry – but I kept off the scales and comforted myself with the thought that, with this extreme action, how could I do anything BUT lose weight?

But on day five, I woke feeling very nauseous, and I couldn't get rid of the feeling all day. By the next morning, this awful, overwhelming feeling of sickness was spoiling everything.

I looked up those websites again.

'A feeling of nausea can often be experienced,' they all said. And then, to my horror: 'Some fasters find that this can last for weeks…'

Weeks?!

I've done so well, I thought. I must try a bit harder. Surely something will make the sick feeling go away? Surely some herbal tea, or exotic fruit?

Nah – I tried everything I could think of, but the sick feeling was ruining my whole day. I was snapping at the children, and kicking the cat. (Metaphorically. Don't worry: I haven't actually got a cat.)

I knew what would make the feeling go away – a piece of wholemeal bread. Something good, healthy, and most importantly, dry and bulky!

Then, I thought – what about something really sensible and nutritious. I had a bowl of Rice Krispies (comfort food!). When that hadn't had the desired instant effect, I made myself a cheese doorstep – with pickle!

Pickle! Oooooh! I hadn't had pickle in years!

The sick feeling hadn't gone – but oh, how I felt happier! Now I tried a Hot Cross Bun. Then I had a packet of crisps. Oh! The carbohydrates! Oh, the naughty, naughty fat!

Next morning, when I awoke to the smell of my eldest son cooking himself a BLT, I asked for one too. I didn't think about what was in it. I didn't even remember that I'm a vegetarian and I don't eat bacon. I just ate.

For elevenses, I had coffee and I demolished that old packet of Rich Tea Fingers that I knew was lurking in the back of the biscuit cupboard.

For lunch I ate pizza. For dinner, I took everyone out to an Indian restaurant and I had a huge vegetable biryani.

It went on like that for a week. I just didn't stop once to think straight.

I utterly lost it.

Of course, when I eventually rediscovered my brain, I was distraught. What on earth had happened to me? And how was I ever going to pull myself together?

I'd fallen off the wagon, and it doesn't half bruise your bum. But bruises heal, and you can climb back on that wagon again! Luckily, I had some expert help. Here's what I learned:

It's so easy at this point to feel really low. Disappointed with yourself. Your self-esteem is in the gutter, because you let yourself down. You failed again.

STOP! You've got to stop thinking like that. That's the first thing Jason said to me – don't treat a negative (falling off the wagon) with another negative (self-blame).

You are not a failure – you're just human.

Even Arnold Schwarzenegger can be knocked off balance! So what if you stuffed all those chocolates? So what if you ate for Britain today? So what if you made an excuse and skived off exercising for a day or two? All is not lost.

Ask yourself now – do you really want to give up – and go back to the old days? Didn't you like the feeling that you were going somewhere, achieving something? Don't let one little blip – or even a big bump – veer you off your chosen path. Remember what you wanted when you first set out on this road. You wanted to get back into those jeans, feel good about yourself, less puffed when you climbed the stairs. You wanted energy to be able to play with the kids. You wanted to wear a bikini.

You made a promise to yourself that you were going to improve your health, fitness and attitudes, particularly towards food and exercise. Those aspirations haven't changed. You still yearn for those things and – hey, look! You're even nearer than you were. You can't possibly give up now.

Falling off the wagon happens to everyone – so don't be upset to have the odd blemish on your chart. Nobody promised that you would be perfect. Life isn't like that. The test of your mettle now is whether or not you can pick yourself up, dust yourself off and get right back on track. Don't think – well, I'll get back on to it tomorrow – do it now! Put the bump in the road behind you straight away.

I know that if one of my small children fell off his bike, I would consider it very important to encourage him to get right back on, even if he's still crying a little. I know that staying off could mean he might give up, maybe forever.

Wouldn't we all say: 'You can't expect to learn to ride a bike without getting a few bumps and scrapes!'

So, if you have fallen off the wagon, get right back on – before you lose your nerve! I did, even after a spectacular fall!

There's another form of falling off the wagon – and you may recognise this about yourself. It wasn't just one thing that pushed you off – not just one lapse. It was more as though you'd let your resolve gradually slip, a little erosion of your ideals bit by bit, day by day, until you realised you really weren't doing anything different at all. No one event sticks out, you've just loosened up the new eating and fitness plan to a point where it is no longer effective.

So do this now:

Retune!

You might be reading this and thinking: 'I don't have to read it all again. I don't need to retune – I know what I want. I know it has to be healthy food. I know the difference between a lettuce leaf and a biscuit.'

But believe me, it helps. I don't know why – but it really does. Maybe you know all these things on a superficial level – but you need to get to the stage where the important messages are second nature, instinctive. And that does take more than simply learning the lesson once. New habits have to be reinforced, over and over again, until your sub-conscious knows them as well as your conscious mind.

Write out in big, bold, red letters your original list of hopes and goals.

Remind yourself why you started, what your feelings were – maybe go through the whole beginning process again.

Write down the small details of what you want, the little things that would mean a lot – like fitting into a particular dress, wearing a bikini on your holidays, walking the kids to school without getting puffed, to lose a stone or two, or to flatten your lumpy stomach!

Pin them up somewhere where you'll notice them all the time – or place them by your bed. Don't let yourself forget.

Now write down some more positive aspirations, things which you can do for yourself every day. So that even if you have a bad time, or some of your ideas go wrong, or you comfort binge, you can still feel you have achieved your positives. They could be: walking the dog, eating some fresh fruit, having an aromatherapy bath, going to the gym or for a run in the park.

Have a think about what might have triggered your fall from the wagon, what might have tempted you to give in to those choccies or have three extra helpings of that lasagne. Avoid the situation where it might happen again. Everyone has triggers that can push them off course, and it is important to know your own.

Keep a list of your trouble spots, and be aware of how to resolve them. If, for example, you have a cocktail party to attend and worry about all of the mini-quiches and dips, fill up on veggies before you go to help keep temptation at bay.

That's why you're keeping notes – not to shame yourself, but to learn where and why you veered off course. And remember to visualise what it will be like fulfilling your aims: shut your eyes and imagine you have achieved your goal and are sunbathing by the pool and feeling fantastic!

Finally, let me identify another hostile force when it comes to losing weight – and that's the diet saboteur.

Never mind you worrying about falling off the wagon. These sinister agents of the devil can actually push you off it.

Diet saboteurs come in all shapes, sizes, genders and relationships. They can be well-meaning mothers, sneaky sisters, catty colleagues, green-eyed friends and even jealous husbands.

Sometimes they don't mean to spoil your good intentions... and sometimes that's exactly what they mean!

I have a work colleague who is always trying to lose weight, like me. She positively preened herself when I came under media attacks about my weight, after I'd been on *Big Brother*. But recently, since I have been noticeably losing weight, she's a nightmare to have lunch with. Because she keeps telling me I look great, and I should stop the dieting now.

'You really mustn't lose any more,' she whines. 'If your face gets any thinner, you'll look scrawny!'

And then she urges me to have a dessert. 'Go on,' she says. 'I am going to. Don't make me eat all on my own. One little profiterole won't hurt. You don't want to become a food bore!'

Now, that's a diet saboteur at her very best. She knows all the little triggers, all the tiny weak prompts that can start a cave-in. Oh, hell, you think... Is my face getting scrawny? Am I becoming a diet bore? And, of course, she's right. One little profiterole won't hurt, will it!

I have now learned how to deal with her. I stick to my guns – but I just say: 'I'd eat it if I wanted to. I just don't fancy it, I'm afraid. But I will have some fruit.'

Her face turns to thunder – and she usually backs down, and doesn't have the profiteroles either!

When you are trying to lose weight, probably the best thing to do is tell no one, unless you really have to. Because so many people hear you're on 'a diet' and see that fact alone as a green light to try their utmost to wreck your plans. It's as though they don't want you to succeed. Mums are different. They do it because they love you, can't stand seeing you 'suffer' and they have a very basic instinct to feed you. Best way to treat them, then, is to stress the fact that you are stuffing yourself full of healthy foods and that you have simply gone off the taste for steak and kidney pie with suet pudding.

Mind you – a word of warning. Watch how you use the word 'healthy' to describe your new eating lifestyle. It can imply that the way Mum cooks is unhealthy!!!

Even those closest and dearest to you can be diet saboteurs. Er, I mean husbands!

You can be full of determination, and excited that you're making great changes when it comes to food, health and fitness, and what does your husband say, or do?

He pooh-poohs the whole idea. He dismisses your fridge full of healthy, fresh, nutritious groceries as 'rabbit food' and scoffs at your resolution to exercise – when what you actually need is a partner who'll join in with you, and not be judgemental.

Unfortunately, partners like that do not grow on trees. If you are lucky enough to have found one – then you are one of the few. If you haven't got one, then you need to be able to shrug aside his negative attitudes, and keep concentrating on your positive ones – or you will too quickly lose the drive to go on.

Sometimes, lack of support from a husband can be annoyingly well-meaning, even loving.

'You're not fat, you're just well-rounded!' he might whisper in your ear, as he comes up for a cuddle.

'You must eat, or you'll be ill!' Mr Anxious.

'That's not the way to do it – try this…!' Mr Know-all.

Or 'I won't like you if you get too skinny!' Mr Control-Freak.

Of course, you know why he is saying those things, don't you?

It's jealousy.

He's worried that you have finally got your act together and you are really going to do it. You're going to be slim, healthy and fit – and that constitutes a threat to how he feels. He probably likes you the way you are now – it makes him feel safe, secure and happy. Think about it. Many husbands – even though they moan about how fat their wives are – don't really want them to look slim and gorgeous. Because A: It'll show them up – if you can do it, why don't they? And B: You might start to be attractive to other men. Whoops! We can't allow that to happen…

Some men feel safe with fat wives because other men don't look at them. He may not know it – it may just be a subconscious fear that you'll leave him if you suddenly become a sexy siren. He won't know how to handle you, how to please you. Or he may just be worried that his safe, comfortable little world will be turned upside down – a fear of the unknown.

Now I'm not suggesting that you turn your quest for slimness and fitness into a psychotherapy session all about him. And please don't turn into a man-hater. But it does help to understand why he may be doing and saying things that ruin your attempts to change your lifestyle.

Because your husband, partner or even best mate, could actually be making you fat! (However, blaming him for all your problems isn't going to help you, either, so let's not even go down that road…)

Change is difficult enough without being undermined by those closest to you. It may seem easier to give in and keep the peace, but that'll only lead to simmering resentment in the long run – and it won't do anything for your self-esteem or health!

So here's what to do:

1. Don't make an issue out of it. To be honest, you don't have to announce to anyone that you're trying to change. If you don't tell your partner you're dieting, he may not notice. You've made a pact with yourself, nobody else.

2. Avoid self-pity. Don't sit in front of a plateful of lettuce moaning about how you would really like to be eating his cod and chips. Feeling sorry for yourself only provokes resentment and no wonder he'll tell you to give up. Eat a healthier version of what he's having – or say you really preferred wholemeal pasta with a simple tomato sauce anyway!

3. Plan ahead. If he brings home a Chinese takeaway, smile, say you had a big lunch and just have a little. Don't make it a problem.

4. Change your way of thinking. You're not on a diet; you're simply looking after your health. So when he presses unsuitable food on you, tell yourself, 'I don't want it,' not 'I can't have it.'

5. If he cooks, and he constantly serves up fried, greasy foods, compliment him on it but limit your portions. Use another excuse to avoid those foods, like you're worried about your skin getting spotty, or you think you might be slightly allergic.

6. Don't upset his routine too much. If you have always cooked huge roast dinners and he likes them, then don't stop – but maybe opt for a healthier way of cooking. Sit the chicken on a rack, instead of in its own juices. Grill, or dry-fry. (A new, non-stick pan or wok can be a slimmer's handiest kitchen aid.) By making little changes over a long period, you'll make enormous differences, without anyone noticing. Treat yourself to a smaller

serving of the main meal and a large serving of vegetables or salad.

7. Identify the source of his fears. If you think he's sabotaging your efforts because he's afraid you'll leave him for someone else, give him constant reassurance. Tell him you're doing this for yourself, nobody else.

8. Explain what's in it for him. By losing weight, you'll be getting back the vitality and energy you used to have, and the enthusiasm for activities you once shared.

9. Don't avoid going out and socialising. You need to have some strategies for coping with eating out. Adopt them religiously so they become habits. After all, there isn't a restaurant in the world that doesn't serve something you can eat. There is always a healthy option – you just have to want to choose it over the rest! Ask for sauces and dressings on the side, so you can control how much you have. But again, don't make an issue of it. And make sure you like what you've ordered, or you'll have a disappointing time when everyone else is enjoying themselves.

10. Treat him by treating yourself. Reward yourself with a new outfit, and wear it somewhere special with him; what about some new lingerie? Remember, slimmers often find their libido wakes up as they lose weight. He'll soon see the benefits of what you're doing!

On the other hand, if he needs to lose weight – you could always try slimming him, too! See Chapter 13 'Slimming your Family' on page 165.

Chocoholism

If you really, really crave chocolate.

If you are the kind of person who has one choccy, and then obsesses about finishing the whole box.

If you find that every single diet and fitness plan you start is wrecked by your love of chocolate...

Then there's a reason – and you've got to find it.

Chocolate has always been linked with love, and many cultures actually believe it to be an aphrodisiac. Casanova found it more effective than champagne with the ladies and the Aztec Emperor Montezuma would drink vast quantities before 'visiting' his 500 wives.

Just think of the famous quotes that exist – just about chocolate:

'Chocolates are not a substitute for love. Love is a substitute for chocolate.'

Or:

'Chocolate is cheaper than therapy and you don't need an appointment.'

And look at what we always give our loved ones on Valentine's Day (or on any other romantic date): chocolates! In studies, women have even said they prefer the stuff to sex!

There's no doubt that we in the Western world view chocolate as a luxury and see it as an expression of love. So do I really have to spell out why you might be feeling a huge need for chocolate? But you don't have to overdo the self-analysis to know that we all need to treat ourselves better, grab a bit of me-time, just generally look after our health both mentally and physically.

Chocolate is your way of patting yourself on the back for a job well done, or comforting yourself during a bad time. So any diet regime that preaches to you 'Thou Shalt Not Eat Chocolate', 'Chocolate Is A Sin' is never going to work for you. What you have got to do is understand why you are craving chocolate, when you succumb and what triggers a scoffing session, and then you have to build your very real need into a new eating and fitness pattern.

We know that chocolate is loaded with calories. But to help me illustrate just how devastating it is for anyone trying to lose weight, let me show you the maths! Now you can see how your efforts can be so quickly sabotaged by succumbing too often:

- For instance, a standard size Mars bar contains 307 calories.
- A Toffee Crisp is 237, a Crunchie 193, a small bag of Maltesers 183, and a Cadbury's Flake 180 – even a fun size Bounty is 141!
- If you fancy a box of Milk Tray – the average sized box, 227 grams, is 1,123 calories.
- A small box of All Gold will cost you 1,078 cals.
- A small box of After Eight (that's 300 grams) will be 1,257 calories.
- The smallest box of Black Magic is 1,035 calories.

You probably need to run over 10 miles to burn off a bar of chocolate. So when we joke that a bar of chocolate goes directly to our hips – we're almost certainly correct!

But all is not lost. You do need to address why you are obsessing about chocolate. Food cravings often stem from basic, un-met needs for fun, excitement or love. Maybe you're under stress, depressed or feeling blue. Do you suffer from too much work and not enough play? Are you tired, with low energy levels – and you convince yourself that chocolate gives you a boost?

Clearly you cannot solve those problems overnight. But you can make a list of the things which do give you a boost; make you feel better; improve your self-esteem – that aren't chocolate.

It could be walking the dog, going shopping, taking a long hot bath, phoning a friend, or finishing that piece of knitting/embroidery/DIY or decorating job that's left half-done. It may sound tame, but it really is a good idea to take up a hobby of some sort – particularly something that needs concentration and uses your hands.

Make yourself keep a chocolate diary – in a little book, which you can keep in your pocket. Get to know when you have these cravings, and why. And what made things better, what successfully distracted you – even if only for a while.

If you are one of those women who crave chocolate particularly before or during your period, remember that diet and exercise are important for you in fighting PMS too. It is best to eat a diet rich in complex carbohydrates (whole grains, fruits and veggies), and to avoid, as best you can, sugar, salt, alcohol and caffeine, before and during your period. Chocolate isn't the only answer.

Above all, remember you are not alone – it's estimated that fourteen out of every ten people like chocolate.

chapter 11

women's problems

No one ever said it was easy being a woman. But that's no reason why we shouldn't have a good moan about it for heaven's sake.

My mate Shirley-Anne and I have been dieting since our teens. Hardly a month goes by when we're not on the phone to each other – no matter where either of us is in the world – having a good old moan about our weight. It's one of the hot topics of our conversation! One week, she's a pound down and I'm asking her for her secret – next week, I'm doing well and she's after mine. It's part of girly bonding, isn't it – to have a good moan about our bodies? It doesn't mean we're obsessed, or that we talk each other down. It's just a girly thing.

We started it the week we left school. SA went to her doctor about her weight – and he gave her one of those drugs we now regard as highly dodgy. It was designed to speed up her metabolism and reduce her appetite. It looked like an enormous, garishly coloured horse pill. In fact, it was strong enough to knock a horse out, as I soon found.

She was losing weight quite well – and then, one day, she forgot to take the horse pill.

'I wonder if I should take two today,' she mused.

'No, don't do that,' I offered. 'I'll take it instead. I could do with losing a few pounds!'

Well, it had the most amazing effect. I was hyperactive for three days. I didn't sleep – at all. I went to bed when my Mum nagged me, but I stayed awake all night, painting, sewing a big, floral flare into a pair of black trousers, reading, and writing in my diary. I was on speed. I never found out whether I'd lost any weight – because I couldn't stay still long enough to stand on the scales.

It was scary. The whole experience frightened us both so much that SA gave the pills back to the doctor. This all happened many years ago. No GP would ever prescribe those things nowadays. Very dodgy!

No, it was far safer, we decided, trying various different diets and then moaning about them. And thus it has been for the past blah-blah years. (Well, about thirty, if you must know!)

However, one thing we have noticed recently about our weight-loss moans – and that's that they've taken on an altered perspective. We're moaning in a slightly different way.

Age has come into the conversation.

'It's so much harder these days,' SA will groan to me.

'I know!' I'll sigh. 'Ten years ago, all I'd have to do is give up breakfast and I could lose half a stone in a week. These days, I starve for a month and can't lose an ounce!'

Age has become a factor in the weight loss saga. And it's awful!

I suppose it's hardly surprising. We women (I've given up caring very much about men, now. They have a section in Chapter 13 – and that's it, I'm afraid!) go through a lot, physically, in the span of one life.

Periods, breasts, PMS, pregnancy, post-natal stress, more pregnancy, menopause, HRT, osteoporosis – the list goes on. (And what, pray tell me, do men go through after puberty and a few wet dreams?)

Our bodies take severe punishment from Nature, right the way through from girlhood to our silver years – so it's no wonder that they react differently to the rigours of dieting, depending on your age.

But why does it appear to become so much more difficult to lose weight as you get older?

It's that old friend, metabolism.

Age makes it slower!

Most women start putting on weight over the age of 35. Scientific research has proved that it is harder to lose weight the older you get because our metabolic rates decline slightly from the age of 25 onwards, which means our bodies burn off calories at a slower rate. This helps explain why nearly 40% of women over 40 are overweight.

Our metabolism gets slower because we lose muscle mass as we age – about a half pound off muscle tissue per year. As we lose muscle tissue, our resting metabolic rate slows. Slower resting metabolic rate equals weight gain. Aaaagh! Less muscle means we grow weaker. Aaaagh!!!

So, as we already know, the single most effective way to sort that one is to do weight training.

Weight training at least twice a week also has another bonus. It helps combat osteoporosis (more about this later). As muscles strengthen, so do the underlying bones.

Our changing metabolism is the main reason that it gets much, much harder to fight the weight battle as we grow older. But there are other factors which don't make it any easier, too.

Stress makes things worse.

As we get older, we women handle more and more stress – whether it's having the babies, managing the family, holding down a career, doing the washing, ironing, chauffering, childminding – or all of that lot together, like me!

Whenever I am asked what I would most like as a gift, I always say 'another eight hours in the day, please!' And I mean it. We women handle a sometimes impossible amount of stress, and stress is a major block to successful weight loss, simply because it raises blood sugar levels and means you're more likely to turn to 'comfort eating'.

Stress activates the fight-or-flight response, the body's involuntary reaction to a threat that makes our hearts pound and our breath shorten. Chief among the hormones released during this response is the stress hormone cortisol. This hormone kicks up your appetite, prompting you not only to want to eat huge quantities, but especially to want sweets and simple carbohydrates – foods that will give you an instant blood sugar spike.

So to combat stress, firstly try to pinpoint what's stressing you out and secondly work at alleviating it.

Build into your day a little 'me' time. If your doctor told you that you must give an extra twenty minutes a day to one of your children – because it was life or death – you would find the time. Try to make yourself a high priority and find the 'me' time from somewhere. Use it to relax, meditate or have some fun. Fun isn't just for kids. Laughing immediately reduces levels of stress hormones in your body.

Take a relaxing bath. Deep relaxation makes you feel calm and refreshed. It is difficult to feel stress when your body is relaxed. Try deep-breathing exercises during which you close your eyes, consciously relax your body and focus on your breathing for five to 20 minutes each day. Try to breathe deeply and remove all other thoughts from your mind.

Exercise actually alters your mood – as effectively as a drug, only legal! It's because it makes your body pump endorphins around your system – the body's own 'feelgood' chemical. Use music, too. It lifts the mood – and that's a proven chemical reaction. Either sit and listen to calming music, or get up and exercise/dance to invigorating stuff!

If you really are badly under stress, don't be shy about consulting your doctor. During a period where I was terribly stressed out, I read a magazine article about it and it gave me the courage to go and ask my GP for help. His response was helpful and encouraging – and I was prescribed Prozac for about six months. For several weeks, I didn't see any change at all in my stress levels. Then, after a while, I realised that I was 'coping' quite well with things that would normally have got me down badly. So don't be afraid. If you need help, go ask for it!

As my Dad used to tell me whenever I got tense: simplify your life, and make sure you are living within your means. Money worries are the biggest cause of stress in this country.

Learn to say no, so that you don't get bogged down with commitments you never wanted. Delegate responsibilities so that you don't end up with all the worries, all the chores. Don't be a workaholic – find a balance.

If you possibly can, stop smoking – it doesn't alleviate stress, it adds to it – cut down on your drink and concentrate on your healthy eating lifestyle change. It will make you feel better within days. And get lots of sleep. Scientists are beginning to discover that sleep deprivation can lead to insulin resistance, a condition some experts think encourages obesity.

Get a massage. Deep-pressure massage stimulates the nerves that cause our levels of the stress hormones cortisol and adrenalin to go down, while the levels of two mood-regulating brain chemicals rise.

Make love. The more we do, the more endorphins our brains release. These 'neuro-hormones' – chemicals released in the brain during exercise and, yes, after sex – are natural painkillers and also help to alleviate anxiety.

Take a walk outside. Direct exposure to daylight stimulates hormones which regulate our natural cycle, so aiding sleep. Stop drinking caffeinated coffee, tea and fizzy drinks, and eating chocolate, before you go to bed. Also avoid alcohol, which is sedating but disrupts sleep.

Make your bedroom dark. Darkness stimulates the production of melatonin, a light-sensitive hormone which again will help sleep.

The Food and Mood Project, run by a British nutrition research group, recently identified 'food stressors' and 'food supporters': foods that make stress worse and those that help. Participants reported that cutting down or avoiding 'food stressors' like sugar (80%), caffeine (79%), alcohol (55%) and chocolate (53%) had the most impact on mental health. So did having more 'food supporters' like water (80%), vegetables (78%), fruit (72%) and oil-rich fish (52%).

Maybe you suffer from Seasonal Affective Disorder (SAD). Sufferers get inexplicably low, miserable and moody in winter months, but positively bloom in the summer. I know one woman who hired a light therapy box (it has to be a special light) and she sits in front of it for several hours a day during the dark months. It has made a huge difference to her life.

I won't pretend that I follow all of these tips – but I do try my best. Over recent years, I have learned to say no to things – like *Big Brother*!

Ah well! I guess I've still got that lesson to learn!

And then, as if we women don't have enough on our plates, we have our own special set of female problems too…

Premenstrual Syndrome is one of those facts of life we girls have to come to terms with very early on. I don't know about you, but I find it very hard to diet at those times, particularly if I am suffering from stomach cramps. I always get the instinctive feeling that eating will help – almost as though I am interpreting the pain wrongly, as hunger. I stuff myself with food, but it doesn't help at all – and then I feel doubly low!

However, the experts say that, while it's tempting to curl up on the couch the minute the PMS mood swings and bloat strike, you'll lose more weight if you exercise during those two weeks before your period. Here's why: the reproductive hormones oestrogen and progesterone are at their peak then and, because they promote the body's use of fat as energy, more fat is burned off when you exercise during this time.

Well, that's the theory anyway – for what it's worth. Just don't preach me that one while I am premenstrual or I'll snap your head off!

Let's look at another woman's problem: the menopause.

I have spoken to many, many women who are trying to lose weight, just at the same time as they are going through some of the most difficult, painful, and distressing symptoms of the menopause.

They all say how much more difficult it is. They exercise, and restrict their intake of food, only to find no change in their body weight, which is even more upsetting.

Doctors say that if you persevere, you will lose weight. It's just that your body is changing, and so are its reactions. Whereas once upon a time, you knew how your body would react to dieting, now you don't. It's a bit like getting to know a new body, all over again.

However, many of the downside elements of the menopause can be alleviated, treated or the risk of them happening to you reduced, by adopting a healthy eating and exercise lifestyle now. It is amazing how many of the charities and self-help groups that support women and conduct the latest research, all come up with the same advice.

Hot flushes – this is the standard advice on how to stop them, from the British Menopause Society:

- Prescription treatments include hormone replacement and other medicines prescribed by a clinician.
- Non-prescription treatments include vitamin E, herbs, foods with soy and effective lifestyle adjustments, such as: regular exercise, cold

showers, decreased stress, cooler rooms and reduced intake of caffeine, alcohol, hot beverages and spicy foods.

What about osteoporosis, where one in three British women find their bones becoming brittle and weak?

By the time we are 30, our bone begins to break down much faster than it can be replaced, a rate which increases each year. During the dreaded menopause, women can lose as much as 50% of their bone mass because levels of oestrogen, a female hormone that has a protective effect on bone, decrease severely.

Many women go on hormone replacement therapy (HRT) to slow down bone loss. But unfortunately oestrogen levels do not naturally go back to their previous levels. As a result, as bone density decreases, the bones gradually lose their strength and become more brittle. If the losses are large, bones can become so weak that they break.

Now, calcium apparently plays the most important role in the development and maintenance of a healthy skeleton. The best sources of calcium come from milk and dairy products, canned fish with bones, tofu, prawns and green leafy vegetables.

To help the body to absorb all this lovely calcium we need to get plenty of the sunshine vitamin: vitamin D. The easiest way of doing this is to go outside and bask in the sunshine for about 10–15 minutes 2–3 times a week. Now how hard is that – but remember to slap on some suncream!

Moving on to heart disease, it is now known that women have three times less risk of heart attacks than men – before they turn 50. However, ten years after menopause, when women are about 60, their risks increase to equal men's risks. Women can protect themselves against heart disease by not smoking, eating a healthy diet and getting exercise.

The same emphasis on healthy diet and an energetic lifestyle is also there in advice on cancer prevention: there is compelling scientific evidence to suggest that overweight or obese women are at an increased risk of cancers of the womb, bowel and kidney. Moreover, women who have been through the menopause have a greater risk of developing breast cancer.

The Department of Health in the UK and the World Health Organisation have reviewed countless scientific studies looking at the link between diet and cancers. In their recent published reviews, both organisations found a link between high intakes of red or processed meat and bowel, breast, lung, prostate and pancreatic cancers.

However, there is good news for the humble fruit and veg: there is evidence from scientific studies that eating plenty of vegetables reduces the risk of bowel cancer; they may protect against stomach cancer and cancers of the mouth, throat and oesophagus; and they may also offer protection against breast, prostate and lung cancer.

In addition, dietary fibre which is found in wholegrain cereals, vegetables and fruit is important for keeping the bowel working normally and may protect bowel cells from cancer too.

And then what about a concern we seem to be hearing more about these days: thyroidism – a dysfunction of the thyroid gland which can make life utterly miserable for women, and a symptom of which is an inability to control one's weight. This from Thyroid UK:

'Exercise is absolutely essential for everybody. There are no excuses! If you have not moved for a long time start by wriggling your toes and shrugging your shoulders – and that is not a joke! You can exercise quite effectively sitting on a chair. For thyroidians, walking is probably the most beneficial exercise.

Eat regularly and sensibly. Do not cut out meals. Do not go on drastic weight reducing diets. For thyroidians, it is particularly important to keep blood sugar levels as stable as possible. What you eat is very important; biscuits and chocolate bars are the worst items as they cause the blood sugar levels to rise and then dip even lower. You need complex carbohydrates: potatoes, pulses, bread, rice and pasta (and it really is so much better if they are brown, wholemeal and unrefined – try buckwheat or millet). Fruit and vegetables are what are needed most.'

Then there's Poly Cystic Ovary Syndrome. You may remember two famous celebs – Posh and Jules (Jamie Oliver's wife) – having PCOS but the fact is that 5–10% of all women are affected by this. Symptoms can be mild or severe from woman to woman; they may have a variety of symptoms including ovarian cysts, irregular periods, high blood pressure, high cholesterol, acne, excess facial or body hair and be overweight or obese. These symptoms get worse over time or with weight gain. You'll be relieved to hear that many symptoms of PCOS can be improved by losing weight through diet and exercising. There isn't a consensus about what sort of diets work best – some experts think that low carb, low fat diets help whilst others would prescribe high fibre, high carb, low fat diets. If you think you have PCOS then you need to talk to your GP about it, and you'll probably be referred to see a specialist who'll be able to prescribe an appropriate set of treatments for you. There's also a great self-help support group that you can get information from – visit www.verity-pcos.org.uk.

Do you see a pattern emerging now? Losing weight and adopting a healthier lifestyle makes a real difference on a number of health issues – it's not just about looking and feeling great, the results are far more long-reaching than that. Pretty convincing, isn't it?

And these are just the health issues concerning women. If you don't want to lose weight and get fit for your own self, your vanity, or your stress levels – then surely you must for the sake of your health.

Reading through all those facts has hardened my resolve even more. Growing older may be something none of us want to acknowledge (I certainly don't! I hated my fortieth birthday and I will most certainly not be celebrating my fiftieth) but I will be looking after this body. Until they invent body transplants, it's the only one I have – and I rather like it nowadays!

Still got your pregnancy weight? Here's how to shift it...

It's one of those times when people can be least helpful if you're overweight – when you've just had a baby.

They say things like: 'You've got to be well-covered if you're breast-feeding,' or, 'You need energy to look after the baby – you can't possibly diet.' To a certain extent they're right – you have got to look after yourself properly. You are tired, and your body has been through a lot.

But at the same time you are a woman and you want your body back. Your man probably wants your body back, too.

And your baby won't mind, as long as he or she has a happy, healthy mother who has the energy needed to look after them and there's a plentiful supply of milk.

Nature invented a brilliant way of returning a mother's body shape – and it's called breastfeeding. *If you can do it*, then it's the best thing you could do not only for baby, but also for you. Breastfeeding stimulates your own stomach muscles to contract, pulling that tummy in naturally. You won't need to do many postnatal exercises if you breastfeed, although you should try to do some.

It also means you are, quite literally, burning oodles of energy to produce breast milk – and then giving it away. You are shedding about 500 calories a day in milk. Most midwives recommend that you don't actually try to lose weight while breastfeeding and that your calorie intake should not fall below 1800 calories a day. Now more than ever, you should eat with the emphasis on feeling healthy, not cutting back on any foods – except the ones we know aren't doing you any good anyway, like refined and processed sugars, starches and carbohydrates.

There are also all sorts of other benefits to breastfeeding – including the fact that it can protect you from certain cancers. So that's tip number one, *if* you can do it.

If you can't – and there are lots of reasons why some mums find it difficult – then keep smiling: there are other ways to give yourself a weight loss boost. I always get very fed up with the prevalent attitude that 'it's easy to breastfeed' or that a woman is selfish if she doesn't.

Take it from me, a mother who has tried it with all five of my babies. I just couldn't get the hang of it, so to speak. In the end, I was always faced with the stark decision – starve my children or give them a bottle.

It annoyed me rather, as I had to work much harder at losing my pregnancy weight than my friends, who all seemed to be more flat chested than I, but much better breastfeeders. They always say size doesn't matter!

My figure zipped back into shape fairly instantly after my first baby. After baby number two, when I had pigged out all pregnancy on ice creams and orangeade, I had two stones to lose.

I was presenting breakfast TV at the time – and couldn't dare turn up on the box two stones overweight. And so the saga continued. With every birth, I put on weight, and never quite lost it all. You don't need to be a mathematician to work out that, by baby number five, things had got a little out of control. If I look at the mother-and-baby pictures in succession, the babies all look quite tiny, but the mother gets larger and more tired!

If you're suffering from a little too much maternal matter, or you're massively motherly, then tackle it now. You will find that a healthier diet will not only lose you weight, slowly but surely, but all the fruits and veggies will give you extra stamina, verve and energy too.

So let's do the sums:

Firstly, how much weight should you put on during a pregnancy? Well, the average weight gain during pregnancy is 25 to 35 pounds. That's between one and a half stone and two and a half stone. During the birth, new mums lose about 12.5 to 14 pounds – about a stone. This leaves approximately 12 to 21 pounds (or a stone or two) of excess weight to be lost in the post-natal period. That's the text book version. Many women put on more weight than that, and it does seem like a huge amount to lose after the euphoria of childbirth passes.

Don't let it get you down. It can be done. But, rather like facing up to the fact that there's a new person in the house, which means a whole new way of living, you have to create a new lifestyle pattern for yourself. Start thinking about you, too. This baby needs a mother who can be fit, active and healthy. Be as disciplined and determined and single-minded about your own health as you are about your baby's.

You wouldn't feed your baby just anything. You wouldn't stuff food inside her. You wouldn't let her eat chocolates and crisps all day. Well, treat yourself the same way. You are as important as she is. She – or he – cannot live without you.

So for the first three months afterwards, focus on healthy eating. When your partner, or mum, asks what they can do to help you – give them a healthy shopping list! Start eating healthily today – you deserve it.

At the same time, develop a realistic exercise plan. One which won't tire you out. One which will build you muscle, because as you now know, the more muscle you have, the more fat you will burn – even at rest!

As you recover, and when your period has returned to normal, try to cut out your unhealthy eating habits, such as snacking on high fat, high sugar foods, midnight feasting and so on.

Make yourself a morning juice, and eat four or five healthy mini-meals during the day. Doing this rather than the usual three meals a day will help combat fatigue, feed your metabolism and burn up fat. Remember to drink plenty of water too – particularly if you are breastfeeding.

By the way, the idea that you should drink milk if you are breastfeeding is a fallacy. You should simply have a healthy, balanced diet – with plenty of fluids.

You will gradually lose weight and regain your figure.

If you gained no more than the recommended 22–30 pounds, it should take you about 4–6 months. For extra weight gained, aim to lose an average of one and a half to two pounds per week.

Start the exercises as soon as the midwife or health visitor says you can – usually about 5–6 weeks after the birth.

I recommend either going along to a specialist post-natal gym session or getting one of the many brilliant exercise videos specially made for new mums. They're better than ordinary exercise videos because they're mindful of the extra pains and strains caused by pregnancy and childbirth – and they also make you do those annoying little pelvic exercises we all forget… and later regret! Many include exercises you can do with your baby, almost using your baby as the weights – babies love this – but do make sure you follow instructions carefully!

Exercise brings physical and psychological benefits, all of which will help if you feel occasionally blue.

Ideally, aim to regularly achieve 30 minutes exercise, per day. Set little goals, like doing 10 minutes of exercise each day and then gradually increase it.

Why don't you buy one of those fantastic jogging pushchairs and go for a run with baby in the park? Or just walk briskly whilst pushing the pram – you'll be surprised at how breathless that can make you!

Just be sure to check it all through first with your doctor or health visitor.

The key is to treat yourself and your body with the same love and respect you have for your baby. Maternal instinct tells us to put baby first – that's why so many mums put on weight but would almost die of embarrassment if their child weighed too much or too little at the weekly clinics. Yet we mums are important, too!

chapter 12

enjoying the journey and dressing for the trip

Imagine you are going on a wonderful holiday – let's say, to Mauritius!

It is going to be perfect. Luxury hotel, perfect weather, lots of sun, sand and sea!

Only one problem – you can't go until, say, six months from now.

That's how you have got to visualise your lifestyle change to a new you. Your new body, your new health, is like a luxury holiday, which you are going to savour and enjoy – because you will have earned it!

But holidays don't just happen. They have to be dreamed about, planned, saved up for, booked. Then the tickets have to be collected, all the paperwork sorted out. Then, when the date gets nearer, there's all that packing (and buying all the stuff you're going to need, like sun cream, insect repellent, toiletries and 300 pairs of knickers) and finally there's the day when you set off. First, a taxi to the station. Then a train ride to the airport. Then all that hanging around and checking in at various desks, before you're finally given your boarding pass, and allowed up the steps to the aircraft.

Even then, your journey isn't complete. There's all the sitting down and wriggling. The steward's safety speech, the drinks trolleys and duty-free sales. The journey does go on and on, doesn't it?

But it's worth it when you get there!

Well, that's what slimming is like. It's brilliant when you get there, but oh – the journey can be long and hard!

One thing, which I really hope I can pass on to you, is something very important that Jason taught me from the very beginning.

The journey (to Mauritius, because that's how we're imagining it!) does NOT have to be hard. In fact, it can be fun, and you should enjoy every moment of it, or you are throwing the time away.

At the very beginning of this book, I mentioned the fact that I used to be a great prevaricator. I would endlessly put things off, until the day (which, of course, never came) when I would be slimmer.

If I was invited out, I would think up lots of excuses, and decline. I would think 'Well, I'll do that another day, when I am looking skinny and fabulous!'

In my job, I have always been so lucky to be asked to glittering parties, showbiz events, film premieres and such. I must have turned down 99% of them, despairing of my figure – and always aware, of course, that there would be a million photographers there.

The truth is, if you go through life turning down such invitations or saying no to exciting events, you are going to miss out.

And if you are like me, having spent much of your life dieting, then you are missing half your life.

And many of those invitations don't come back again, no matter how you hope!

Anyway, what's to be ashamed about? So you're larger than you want to be. It doesn't mean you have to lock yourself indoors! There are fantastic clothes around nowadays to fit any size. Dawn French is a plus-size but she always looks fantastic, and sexy.

It is important to value yourself now, and not just when you are slim. If you think you are only worth being with when you're slim, then you're buying into the very worst sort of values that, I'm afraid, are bandied about by our figure-conscious media.

There are lots of mistakes made, though, when it comes to choosing clothes for the larger figure.

In fact, it's something I gave a lot of thought to when I was preparing to go into the *Big Brother* house, as I knew that my larger figure would fall well and truly under the media spotlight.

My friends and I carefully studied old tapes of past *Big Brothers*. I would be seen from top to toe, all the time. There was a lot of sitting down, on low, uncomfortable-looking sofas. That would mean my middle would be permanently scrunched up – not a very flattering pose.

Many of the shots were taken by cameras hidden in the ceilings, and that gave everyone a slightly compressed look – terribly un-flattering except for the tall and lean Goldie.

So I made up my mind that I wouldn't commit the common sin, made by a great many overweight women. I wouldn't wear clothes that were already tight, or even close-fitting. It would look as though I was trying to cram too much in. I'll go for loose-fitting clothes, I thought.

But I overdid it, I can see now. I bought such large, voluminous tops and jackets that I resembled a walking tent. What did one of those rather nasty headlines say about me? Oh yes, I remember it well – 'Big Blubber!'

Those big, roomy outfits didn't make me look slimmer – they made me look larger than I actually was (which was bad enough!).

And there's another thing. If you are overweight, it's no good simply opting for the bigger sizes at high street stores.

I bought a size 20 jacket, and it dwarfed me – not because it was too big (in fact, I couldn't do the buttons up) but because it was made for a much larger lady, someone who was a correctly proportioned size 20. Tall and well-built. You know, an Amazon! Well, that wasn't me! I am only five feet and five inches. I'm pretty short – but I was rounded! I need a size 12 jacket with more room inside it!!!

One of my other huge mistakes was a sort of artist's smock, which I thought was beautiful on the peg, but which ballooned on me, and really did smack of the kaftan look of the 1970s.

It was the first thing most people mentioned when I came out of the *Big Brother* house.

'Why on earth did you wear that smock thing so much?' they asked.

Looking back on the videos, I looked better in simpler lines, like a simple jumper with trousers, instead of trying to camouflage my bulges with lots of layers and folds.

So I'd recommend going to a shop which specialises in making clothes for overweight people – that way, they'll be correctly proportioned and you won't end up wearing a jacket where the intended waistline is flopping around your bum. You need to understand your shape – even if the long-term intention is to lose it!

It's important to get the clothes right – because you deserve to look good and feel confident, no matter what size you are. It's vital to enjoy every stage of the journey.

It's also vital that you learn to love your body now. It's a sad fact that most women in this country hate their own bodies. I know I did.

Well, it's the only one you've got – and actually, as long as you are healthy and physically able, then you have no worries. Because, with enough hard work and determination (notice I didn't say willpower), you can change it into a body shape that you really love.

You won't need willpower. I didn't. In fact, I have very little willpower.

The only thing you need is something I hope I have been able to explain throughout this book. You need knowledge (about the true qualities of food and the true benefit of a little daily exercise), understanding (how these facts can bring about a real change in you) and belief (that you can do it!).

So learn to love your body now – the more you love it, the quicker it will lose that excess weight. Now is the time to dress it well, so that you won't make the mistakes I made on *Big Brother*.

For the very best advice, I thought I'd check out what they say at one of Britain's most influential high street stores, Marks and Spencer.

When you think of it, M&S were probably responsible for one of the worse fashion faux pas for British women with a weight problem – the baggy T shirt and leggings look.

At the height of those awful leggings years (the late 1980s), it was reckoned that a million pairs of stretch black or blue leggings, size 18 or over, were sold in this country every day! A shamefully high proportion of those came from Marks and Spencer, who lovingly called them ski-pants, but which looked distinctly un-sporty when strutting behind a pushchair, under a big, baggy sweatshirt with a floppy old pair of trainers to finish off the look. What on earth made us think we looked acceptable?

Truth is, I think we wore them because they were comfortable. We didn't think nearly enough that, for the overweight woman, it was never a flattering look.

'Well, we've come an awfully long way since then!' laughs Louise Salt, one of the product developers at Marks, and the lady most responsible for designing their new 'plus' range.

Louise is responsible for what actually appears on the store shelves and hangers. She has to work closely with the clothes designers, as she is the essential liaison point between customer and provider.

'We've come to realise that larger ladies want to look every bit as trendy as slimmer ones – it's just that they need clothes with more thought applied to the design.'

I had a little moan at her about that size 20 blue jacket which I had taken into *Big Brother* with me. I'd bought it so that it would look smart, and loose. But when I wore it on TV, I found that, from the back, you could see the natural waistline of the jacket flapping around my bum.

To buy a jacket that was loose enough around the arms and chest, I had been forced to buy something that was essentially cut for a gargantuan woman, twenty feet high.

'Why don't you guys ever design for women who are short, fat, round and tubby?' I demanded. Just because I have grown rounder, it doesn't mean I have gained several inches in height!

'We do, nowadays,' she replied, ushering me towards a rail with some very yummy garments on them.

'Just look at what can be achieved with a little extra thought,' she smiled. 'But just think – British ladies come in all varieties and shapes. What may be a good fit for you may not flatter the next large lady. You have got to learn what your shape is, and then you will start to understand how to dress it in the best way.

'That's why we have had to do three different lengths in trousers, two different lengths in skirts and even two choices of length in long cardigans!'

The first and most important lesson to be learned, according to the top designers, is getting the underwear right.

High street stores like Marks and Spencer have at last come to the realisation that those of us with big boobs aren't necessarily big all around the back, and vice versa. In other words, they are selling big back/small cup

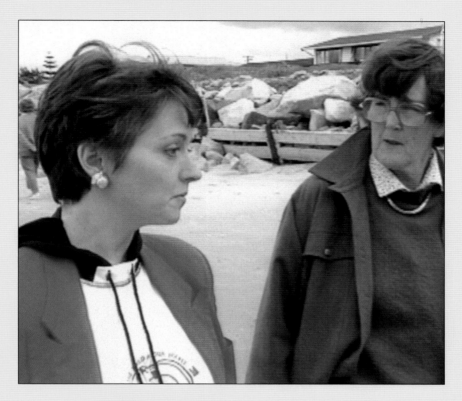

This shot was taken on Waihi Beach in New Zealand, during my filming of a documentary about cot death (I am interviewing the cot death expert here, Dr. Shirley Tonkin). By this time I was losing control of my weight (possibly for understandable reasons, since the death of my child) and all I could fit into was a baggy old jacket and leggings. I look back now and can see that it was then that the weight started to pile on. Of course, my appearance was the last thing on my mind – but maybe that was when I started "comfort eating".

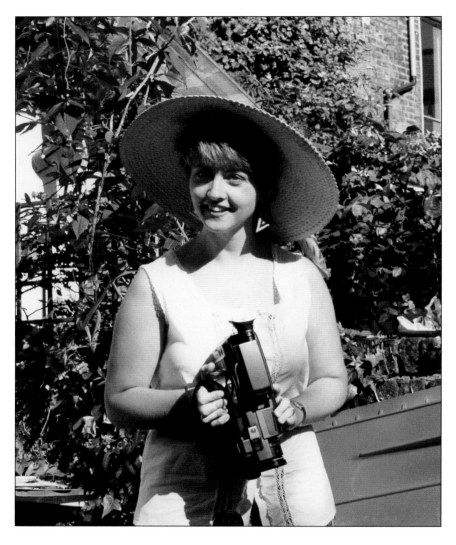

When I was researching the pictures for this book, I was astonished to see how little I featured
in any of my home photos. This picture shows why. At some point after the birth of my first son,
I became the family photographer – and hid behind the camera on many occasions. If ever someone
else offered to take a photo – and it was a rarity – I would hide myself behind assorted children.
Despite my profession, I had become decidedly camera-shy!

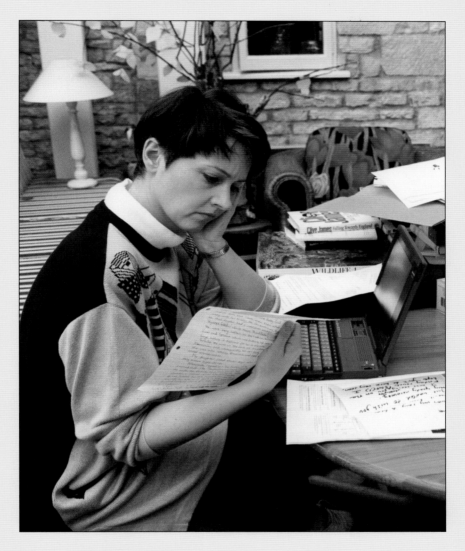

Here I am at work, writing and researching my various books and columns. I am currently working on two novels and a cookery book for children! These days my life is very sedentary – much of the day is spent sitting down and writing, which I love. The trouble is, it is just too easy to pop into the kitchen and grab something to eat and drink. Take a look at the enormous baggy jumper too – I thought it hid my weight well, but actually it just made me look bigger!

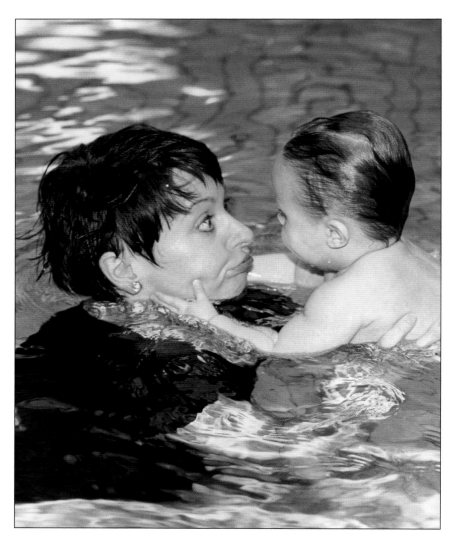

This shot was taken a couple of years ago, to publicise my column in *The Sun* newspaper. "Let's see you swimming with the children," they said. I think they would have liked a full frontal shot of me in a swimming costume – but no way! I donned a black T-shirt and kept my body well under the water!

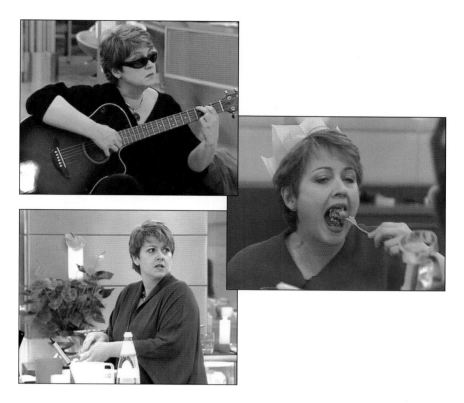

Me in the *Big Brother* house. Although my participation generated masses of hurtful and abusive press in the nation's tabloids, the experience actually marked the start of something new and positive for me. It was the turning point for my becoming The New Me. I have never looked back since.

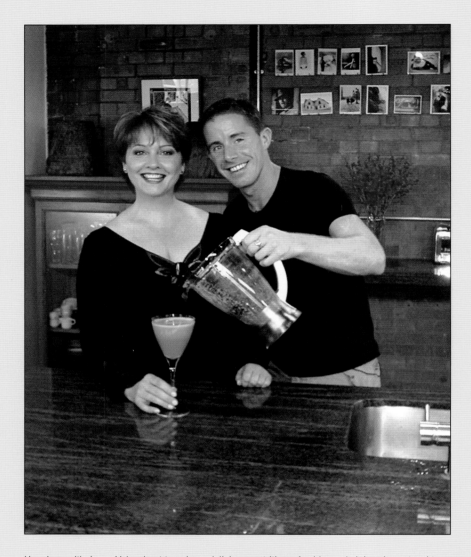

Here I am with Jason Vale, about to enjoy a delicious, nutritious, freshly-made juice. Jason taught me that there was a new way to lose weight – without dieting, without denial and most importantly without self-hatred. I couldn't have done it without him.

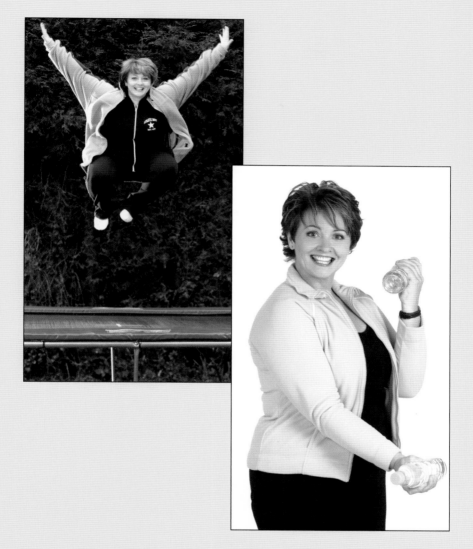

If you're trying to lose weight, exercise is absolutely vital. Find something you enjoy doing and it won't be such an effort – trust me! I love trampolining – not only does it keep me fit, but it's great fun to do too. And don't forget about weight training either – even simple weights like these water bottles will make a difference to your muscle tone and general health, as well as helping to boost that old favourite, the metabolism.

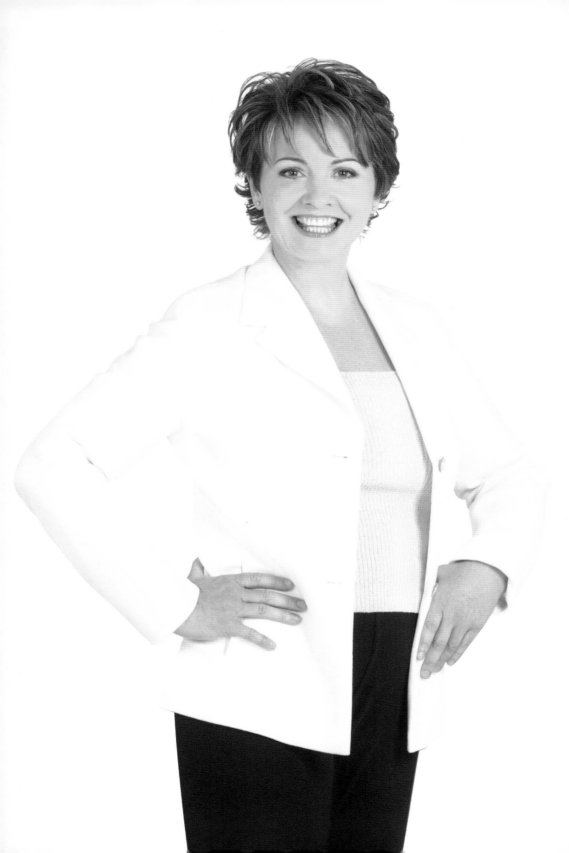

and small back/big cup bras. They are also understanding that larger ladies can also want to wear sexy strings instead of big knickers.

So there's really no excuse not to be loving that body straight away – although I still don't know whether I will ever have the courage for a 'string'!

So here are some top tips for a New You look, gleaned from the experts (not me!) on how NOT to look like I did on *Big Brother*!

1. Don't be afraid to try anything – if you've always wanted to wear a mini skirt then try it. Just spend a lot of time in front of the mirror to make sure you've got the look right! Ask an honest friend to come along and give you her opinion.

2. Good staple items that should be in any larger lady's wardrobe: go for a layered look; a simple tunic top (patterned but not with horizontal stripes, or plain), combined with dark elasticated waist trousers and topped off with a long cardigan, shirt or jacket.

3. Don't buy clothes that are too big! Don't fall into the trap of thinking that the more fabric there is, the more flab you'll hide. It can even make you look bigger. Clothes should touch you comfortably all around!

4. Patterns: Do not wear head to toe large prints as this can make any shape or size seem bigger. Break a print up, by combining with a plain top or bottom. Small prints like a tiny floral design or spot can be OK top to toe, though.

5. Colours: Many larger ladies feel conspicuous in bright colours – but you must choose a colour to go with your personality, not your size. If you do go for something bright, maybe team it up with a more neutral colour, so that the overall effect isn't overpowering.

6. Black and white: Yes, it is true that black and darker colours are

slimming. What about white? Can larger ladies wear white outfits? It depends entirely on the mood. White linen apparently sells very well in the summer, even in the very large sizes. Be wary – just try it and see if the look suits.

7. Don't put off buying new clothes until you are slim. Enjoy clothes now. There are lots of elasticated waists in skirts and trousers which will see you through two or three sizes, as you lose weight. Also, a fitted shirt can be worn later as an overshirt.

8. Accessorise – scarves add to the layered look and can be very complimentary as they can hide double chins, and flabby tops of arms. Pashminas are great at this, too. Don't be afraid of belts – they can be worn as an accessory rather than pulled too tight.

9. Frills – too much fuss will make you look frumpy and even add to your size. They can also draw the eye to a part of the body you may not want. Keep to softer, simpler but distinct lines.

10. Finally – some tips on the styles of clothes which are most flattering to the plus-size shopper:

   Trousers – go for a bootleg cut, not wide all the way down. Make sure they are long enough!

   Tops – V necks and wide crews are more flattering than simple round necks.

   Jackets – make sure they're long enough to cover your bottom, and no double breasts, please!

   Skirts – bias cut are more flattering. Knee length or long. If you want to wear minis, make sure you've got the right legs for it!

   Dresses – bias cut is best, go for a long length and wear heels to give you some extra height!

Remember too that most high street stores are flexible, you can return or exchange items that you're not happy with – because you know what it's like, sometimes you're desperate to do some retail therapy and you buy something that felt oh so right at the time... but when you get home you think, oh, the colour is wrong, the shape is wrong, or your children and partner hate it. At least you know you can go back to customer services and return the clothes or exchange them without feeling guilty about it.

It's amazing really, isn't it – that high street stores have only just come around to understanding how to dress their fastest growing consumers! They reckon that one in four women in the United Kingdom is a size 20 and above. According to the World Health Organisation, on a global scale, women are getting larger every year! The average size of a British woman in the 1960s was 34-24-33. By the 1980s, the average lady was 35-26-37, and in the year 2000, 36-28-38. So there's no shame in it. But I do think there's room for action – because I bet most of those women would really like to be a size 12.

I just hope that if you are one of those people, then this book will help you start the journey to a new you – whatever your size or shape now. The important thing is to feel happier in your whole outlook.

Envisaging my 'dieting' as a journey has made it more fun. When I lost the first stone, I thought, 'Mmmm. I've booked the tickets to Mauritius.'

With the next few pounds, I was able to feel I'd started packing my holiday suitcase.

At a stone and a half, I was at the airport.

Jason would ring me and ask: 'Where are you now?' and I'd reply: 'I'm sitting in my seat, and the stewardess is bringing round the drinks!'

'Orange juice only, remember!' Jason would laugh.

It got to be really exciting, especially when the captain ordered 'cabin doors to manual!' and we started the descent into Mauritius airport.

Right now, I can honestly say I am still on my holiday, and it is fabulous.

It is everything I wanted it to be. I feel fit and energetic, and I like passing by in front of mirrors – I still can hardly believe it's me.

I've come a long way – and this time, I think I'm staying!

chapter 13

slimming your family

1. Men and weight: the facts

Obesity levels are soaring – a report from the charity Weight Concern reveals that rates have trebled in the last 20 years; obesity now affects about 20% of the UK population and over half of the population is overweight. According to a government report on obesity, in Britain 18% of men are clinically obese, compared to 21% of women. And 61% of men are officially overweight, compared to 57% of women. For the first time, the number of overweight men in the UK now exceeds the number of overweight women.

Dr Campbell, an obesity expert in the UK, says inactivity is one of the main reasons for the rise in obesity. He says: 'Forty years ago the average man would walk the equivalent of a marathon a week. Today's man hardly does a thing.' This problem is also even more worrying in our children. Many no longer walk to school, most children (notably boys) watch the television or computer screens for hours every day and few do regular sporting activity.

But back to our partners for the moment. If you think your man needs to lose a bit of weight, then read on…

If you imagine your partner might go to a slimming club, then forget it: fewer than one in 100 men go to slimming clubs (which is why Dr Campbell has launched a weight loss programme specifically for men on the internet site www.fatmanslim.com. It's well worth a look).

Your partner could be a ready made 'diet buddy' for you. It makes sense. After all, you are trying to embrace a whole new lifestyle – one which is going to dictate what food is in the fridge, what goodies are in the pantry. In fact, you are going to redefine what is a 'goodie' – so it would help if your partner were in on the act.

But what will he think of the idea?

Firstly, be careful how you broach the subject. Remember, men have feelings too – and they are just as likely to react the way you would, if your husband just announced to you one day that you needed to lose a few pounds.

If he hasn't even thought about it – or if he really thinks he is Brad Pitt – then tread carefully. Stress to him how you think the whole family should be more health-conscious and that you need some active support. Would he come along to the gym with you?

However, most men are like us – we are bombarded with media images of how we should look, and feel ourselves falling short of that ideal.

He may be looking for that extra little push from you. And he may be flattered that you'd like his help.

But agree on the rules first. No judging each other. There's nothing more likely to send you back to the biscuits and potted noodles than a man who feels he has just been given licence to criticise your shape. Equally, you must not nag him. Just try to both be enthusiastic about getting a little fitter, a little healthier. Stress to him that he will still be able to have a curry and a beer with the lads. Men have a morbid dread of diets!

But he and you do need to understand that men have different hurdles to clear when they are dieting. For a start, men should eat more than women and – this is unbelievably unfair – they can often get away with less exercise.

I know that on this healthy eating plan we are not talking about calorie counting, fat grams or 'points', but it might help you to know that, officially, men need to stick to 2000 calories a day and exercise for about 20 minutes, three times a week, if they want to lose weight.

So expect him to eat a higher volume of food than you. But it should still all be healthy, whole food.

Ten ways to help your man get in shape

1. Realise it's your problem too

Men are notorious for neglecting their health and few see their GPs unless forced to by their partners. Dr Campbell says: 'Women are the driving forces behind men's health. Men often aren't as bothered about their weight as women and won't do something about it until they are told they have a health problem, like high blood pressure. It's up to women to take the initiative.' Do be subtle though. Men can become very stubborn if they think they're being nagged. You'll get the best results if he thinks it was all his idea.

2. Work out how overweight your man is

Chances are you'll be able to guess by the bulge of his belly, but working it out scientifically will give him the best goal to work towards. It may also hit home that it is a serious problem which needs to be tackled.

Calculate his Body Mass Index (BMI) by dividing his weight in kilograms by his height in metres (e.g. 98kg divided by 1.8m = 54.44) Then divide the result by the height in metres again (e.g 54.44 divided by 1.8m = 30.2). This total is his BMI. If the BMI is under 25 then he's perfectly fine; 25 or greater and your man's health is considered to be overweight. A BMI of over 30 is obese and over 40 is severely obese.

3. Measure his waist

It's vital to measure his waist as the risk of coronary heart disease increases if it's over 94cm (37 inches). Carrying fat in this area is linked with the furring-up of arteries that causes heart problems. Men typically put on weight around the waist. Current research shows that the average man's waistline measures 38 inches – 2 inches more than it was 20 years ago. It has been estimated that by 2020 this figure will increase to 40 inches.

Measure your bloke's waist one centimetre below the belly button when he has just breathed out slowly. Check he's not holding his belly in.

4. Lead by example

It's always easier to lose weight if there are two of you. Make a joint pact to get fit together. Don't order him to do 50 press-ups while you lie on the sofa. Find activities that you enjoy doing as a couple.

Dr Campbell says: 'Women need to be positive for their men rather than focusing on the negative. They need to make it clear they are sensitive rather than judgemental.'

5. Make low fat food taste good

Reduce saturated fats in what you eat (that is, cut down on full fat dairy products and get him to trim the fat off his steak and chops) and cut out all snack foods immediately (bin the pies, crisps, biscuits and cakes). Fill up on fruit and vegetables and use spices and herbs to give a richer taste to low fat foods.

6. Forget counting calories

You both have to be realistic otherwise you'll still be in the same position this time next year. Ideally your man should take in 500 fewer calories per day to lose weight. But how many of us know how much 500 calories is?

Dr Campbell says the best way to lose weight is to reduce what you eat in one day by one-fifth.

7. Make sure he eats breakfast – but not a fry-up

Breakfast will power him until lunch and help fight the mid-morning urge to snack. Encourage him to eat cereal or toast with low-fat spread (not butter). He should eat regular meals, filling up on high fibre carbohydrate foods (wholemeal pasta, baked potatoes, brown rice, wholegrain bread, wholegrain cereals) and cutting down on sugar and fat. Get him hooked on juicing in the morning – that way he'll benefit from those vital vitamins and minerals and, if you play your cards right, he might even wash up the juicer afterwards!

8. Get moving

There's no point joining a gym with the intention of sweating it out three times a week if your man has no intention of going. The golden rule is to improve your activity levels on a daily basis – put simply, get moving!

Dr Campbell says: 'We have such sedentary lives nowadays so you have to take every opportunity to be active. Get off the bus stop one stop early and walk. Walk to the local shop rather than take the car. Or park at the far end of the supermarket car park. It all adds up and makes a difference.'

9. Get your man to cut down on alcohol

Alcohol contains calories; excess calories over a long period of time without exercising will inevitably mean weight gain.

Try to encourage him to drink less, as it might be impossible to persuade him to avoid alcohol altogether. Remember it's a habit, too. Simply getting used to drinking less will work wonders over time. It's better for his heart as well!

Diet drinks might help the calorie intake – and at least they're better than the high-sugar beverages. But better still is to try to replace the ritual of going out and drinking with something else – say, a trip to the cinema or theatre – or get him to take up a sport or new hobby. Better still, take up a new hobby together!!

10. Get him to read this chapter

There's only so much you can do for him – he has to do some work too!

Now, let's look at the food he can eat, without your man worrying about having to eat too much 'rabbit food'.

I've tried to tailor some of these points with men in mind. But of course, men are all very different. I know some who would rather die than give up their pie and chips. I know others who talk about health and weight almost as much as me.

So here goes, with just a few ideas:

1. Both of you should get used to drinking plenty of water before and during every meal: it'll fill you up, help you eat smaller portions and aid your metabolism.
2. Stop eating 'man-made' carbs after six pm: baked potatoes and rice are OK – but not bread or pasta. This really works! I bumped into Jono Coleman at a 'do' the other day – and he has lost lots of weight. He says the single most important tip he could pass on to others was this one.

3. Fill wholemeal sandwiches with loads of salad and chicken instead of cheese, coleslaw or dressings. Those sarnies will still look man-size – but they'll be much healthier.

4. If you want to eat chips at home, cook the real thing. Cut potatoes up into big chunks, put on a lightly greased baking tray, spray a little olive oil over them and bake for about 15-20 minutes until cooked.

5. Dry-fry lean mince for chillis or bolognaises. Drain any fat off before adding fresh herbs and chopped tomatoes. He may be used to the taste of oily, fatty ingredients, but the taste of fresh vegetables is just as potent, especially with herbs. Add some chillies too – there is a theory that spicy food boosts the metabolism!

6. Go for low fat options when you buy foods – low fat yoghurts rather than Greek, low fat cheeses, healthy eating products. Just check the labels to ensure they're low in additives too.

7. Cut down on sugary drinks. Go for trendy bottled water when you're out – or just a glass or two of wine. Wean yourself and him off sugar in your coffee or tea. Then later on, try weaning yourself off the coffee and tea – because you want to eventually give up drinking caffeine! Try to use the lowest fat milk you can.

8. If you are going out with your mates for a curry, pick a tandoori dish rather than a creamy curry. Have roti bread rather than naan bread and go for boiled rice instead of pilau.

9. Eat plenty of vegetables. They fill you up and are healthy too.

10. Remind him that he can eat and drink more and still lose weight if he exercises.

2. Children and weight: the facts

When we're talking about weight loss, there's one extra and very important factor we women must learn to deal with – and that's the growing epidemic of obesity among our children. Recent studies show that one child in nine is obese. In as little as five years, that figure is projected to rise to a shocking one in five.

Many of us are mothers, and we have got to learn how to help our children be fit and healthy – not fat, lazy couch potatoes as so many are.

The problem is – and I have a great many concerned letters about this coming in to my column in the *Daily Mail* – we may want to stop them becoming fat, but we also want to stop them from becoming obsessed with body image and the insane, media pressure to be thin. It's a real dilemma.

When I first started in broadcasting, some 25 years ago, the hot topic for discussion was always anorexia. Later, with Princess Diana's astonishing and courageous honesty, we also learned about bulimia – and the fact that these eating disorders can crop up anywhere, even in the 'nicest' of families!

Those concerns are still there. In fact, you could argue that a generation of fat, sedentary children is yet another symptom of malnutrition or food abuse. It's yet another eating disorder.

So it is important to deal with the problems of children overeating as sensitively as those who under-eat.

I have a very close friend whose son was getting very large around the middle – a Billy Bunter type of child. He used to joke about it, but inside, we knew he was hurting.

Then, when he grew a little older and passed into secondary school, you could tell he was being bullied about his weight.

My friend and I talked and talked about what she should do. In the end, she took what I think was the best possible course. Wimbledon was coming up – and she waited for everyone in the family to take an interest in the play on the TV screen. Then she announced that she had enrolled the whole family (husband, son plus two older daughters) for membership at their local racquets centre.

It worked very well. Within weeks, all the family were regulars. She and her husband became fitter as they encouraged the children to explore all the amenities, the squash courts, the table tennis, the gym and the pool.

Her son was never made to feel that he was being 'slimmed' or given any preferential treatment at all. He merely joined in with the whole family.

Over a year, he must have lost over a stone in weight – and is much fitter. They all are – even the daughters, who at first thought it was a real drag.

Nutrition is probably something best tackled as a family issue too. You cannot expect to lecture a child about not eating crisps and chocolate bars if the rest of the family is doing so. An overall approach is needed. In other words, now is the time for the whole family to revise their eating habits.

To avoid power struggles over food, don't have the bad choices around! Yes, I know that children's TV is a non-stop barrage of adverts for sticky, gooey, sugary sweets, but it doesn't mean they have to be on offer at home. Get the fruit bowl out and keep it topped up with the things your child especially likes.

Increase the activity level of the family. Think about how many family activities these days are sedentary: computer games, television, dining out. Create opportunities to promote exercise, such as taking a family bike ride or even a family jog. You'll all feel better.

Quietly observe and try to find out when and why your child turns to 'comfort' food or when and why they snack. There may be an underlying problem you should be dealing with that has nothing to do with food.

But above all, focus on health goals instead of talking about physical appearance. Try not to make your child feel that he or she doesn't look right. Emphasise the health benefits of exercise and physical fitness, including how great it feels to be strong and active (for more ideas of incorporating fitness into your family lifestyle, see the section on fitness for the family – chapter five).

Above all, remember that you also have to be a role model, a good example. It's hard work, but it will be worth it for you and your child.

chapter 14

living the life I want to lead

The other day, Jason and I were planning a new workout routine for a video we're making. We'd just done the ten minute routine twice through – and I was quite pleased to see that he was breathless and sweating profusely.

I knew *I* was, but I had thought that was just because it was me, and I'm about as fit as a box of snooker balls compared to Jason, who's all muscle and bottled enthusiasm.

We both slumped down on sofas, and glugged away at our ever-present water bottles.

Then I confessed.

'Do you know,' I remarked, 'that even after all the hard work I have done to change my eating lifestyle – and after all that exercise we've just finished – I could still kill for a piece of chocolate, or a glass of Bacardi and coke?'

It was true.

We were chatting away so pleasantly, with the morning sun streaming in through the window and the music playing softly in the background. Somehow, though, it would have seemed even more relaxing if I'd only had a glass of something bubbly, and I was sipping it as we spoke. The bottle of healthy water just didn't fit the same bill.

Why oh why did I still feel that, after all this time?!

Truth is, I only wanted that drink, or the morsel of chocolate, because I have been conditioned over so many years to believe that it's what I needed at the time – and even now that still affects me.

We're all conditioned to think this way.

For instance, consider this: You've had a rotten day at work, it rained all the way home, the heel snapped off your shoe and you got splashed by a passing car. You put your key in the door, your wet things on the hallstand, you kick off what remains of your shoes and you go to the kitchen.

What I need is a stiff drink, you think.

So you pour yourself a gin and tonic or a glass of wine, and you go and slump in front of the TV. You take a sip, lean back into the cushions and say 'Aaah! Now *that's* relaxing!'

But wait! There hasn't been a long enough period of time for the alcohol in that drink to have even reached your bloodstream, let alone cause a chemical reaction.

You see, it's not the drink that has relaxed you – it's the sitting down and nestling back into the sofas. You have just associated the two sensations for so many years that you think it is the drink that has this wondrous effect. But it isn't.

The conditioning is very strong, though. You see it everywhere in advertising, and in the behaviour of ourselves and those around us.

'What you need is a strong drink,' we say to people who are too stressed out.

'Have a chocolate – you deserve it,' we say on Mother's Day, or birthdays, or even when we visit someone in hospital.

Yet what do chocolates, or even drinks of alcohol, really do?

They simply make you want another one.

It happens to me with packets of crisps. Just one packet of crisps cannot hurt, I think. Yet I find it almost impossible to have just one packet of crisps. The only thing they ever make me want to do is have another.

And that is what is wrong about so many of the foods that we as a society have come to like. So many of them are processed and contain refined sugars and flours – which are basically just there in order to lengthen their shelf life.

I had it all explained to me once by a miller. I was on a school trip to one of those beautiful working mills somewhere in the Midlands.

No, it wasn't that long ago. I wasn't one of the schoolchildren. I was a Mum, dragged along for the trip by a harassed geography teacher who needed all the help he could get.

Anyway, this miller showed me two bags of flour. One was white, refined flour. The other was wholemeal.

'If I left those bags in the corner of the room,' the miller went on, 'after a few weeks, that bag of wholemeal flour would be crawling with weevils.

'The bag of white flour would just be sitting there, unchanged.'

And why?

Because the wholemeal flour is packed with fibre, vitamins and minerals, which are healthy and to be enjoyed by us, by weevils – or by any other bug, mouse or rat! The refining process takes away most of those things and in fact by law nowadays, the flour industry has to add back in certain amounts of calcium, iron, thiamine (vitamin B1) and niacin (vitamin B3) to refined flours. Whole grain and wholemeal flour naturally contains these vitamins and minerals, and a whole lot more besides.

Isn't it crazy? No wonder the weevils go for the brown sack!

If we had any sense, we would too. But the one thing the weevils have better than us is that they don't watch the TV or read magazines, and they're not subjected to the advertising hype which would be telling them to go for the white sack. Instead, they go for the stuff that smells like living, healthy, nutritious food.

There's another thing, though. Processed and refined foods are low in fibre – which means that they are digested quickly, leading to a rapid rise and fall in your blood sugar. The body doesn't like peaks and troughs in its blood sugar levels. It likes to keep those levels... well, er, level.

So it rushes in a load of insulin, to bring things back down to an even plane.

The insulin kicks the excess sugar out – but where can it deposit all that unwanted stuff?

In your fat cells, that's where.

And that's why eating lots of refined foods can make you fat.

But, oh dear, it doesn't just stop there, either.

Because after a sugar high, you tend to experience a sugar low. So you get hungry faster and you therefore want to eat more. The upshot of this is, not only have you eaten one packet of crisps and a doughnut – but you are almost bound to eat another!

Let's go back to my still wanting, occasionally, to kill for a piece of chocolate or a drinkie.

Jason says he used to be fat, eat all the wrong things, and drink beer. Now, he doesn't ever want to.

I don't know whether I will ever make the 100% change that he has been able to do. I don't even know whether I want to. But I do know this – a little knowledge can be life-changing.

It's like the sausage. You remember the sausage from chapter one? Once you know what's in it, you simply lose the appetite for it. Now, I do not think I will ever be quite so touchy about the odd piece of chocolate, or indeed the odd drink. But I do know now that, when I crave something sweet – usually in the early evening – I recognise it for what it is.

I know it is simply a craving for sugar.

I have found that understanding that means I can make a much more rational decision.

Often, I go to the fruit basket instead. I love pineapple – and there's no doubt that a couple of slices of pineapple makes the craving go away.

A drink doesn't.

I always end up having another.

A piece of chocolate doesn't.

I always end up having another.

It's like magic – except it's a sort of dark, sinister magic. It's oh, so easy, to be seduced by the dark side!

But I have made a change in the way I eat, and the way I exercise, and the way I live my life.

My kitchen is always full of fresh fruit and vegetables – it looks like a greengrocer's. And before you whinge about the price of fruit and veg – it really isn't more expensive than buying processed, ready-made, prepared stuff, especially if you buy fruits and vegs that are in season. You can even bag some brilliant bargains at the end of the day in the market, if you're lucky enough to have one near you.

But, it is more time consuming. I find I am doing a lot more cooking than I used to – and that is very difficult, if you are overworked, underpaid and stressed out already, as so many of us are.

When Jason first told me to start juicing, especially in the morning, I told him: 'I don't have enough time to do that in the morning – you ought to see how busy I am first thing, what with four children to get to school!' Etc., etc.! Oh, I did give him an earful!

But the real truth is that it hardly takes a minute now to make a juice, because I've made it part of my morning routine. It hardly takes five to make a smashing, healthy, nutritious soup. A tuna salad takes about three minutes. A chicken stir-fry about ten.

Eating healthily is only a problem if you really want it to be.

The difficult bit is changing your mindset. Once you've done that, the rest follows quite well.

Of course, I did lose a lot of weight once before – about four years ago, just after my divorce. I think I did it as a reaction to what was going on in my life. I embarked on a rigorous exercise routine which was, looking back, impractical and impossible to keep up. I practically starved myself for weeks at a time, and then binged out on rubbish. I never addressed the true concern, which was: *why had I put on all that weight in the first place?*

So, when I reached my target weight, I went out to dinner to celebrate – and started, very quickly, to put all that weight back on. When I next saw myself in the mirror, I was mystified.

Where had all that weight come from? Why had I so easily put it all back on again?

I was honestly, truly puzzled.

But now I know.

My relationship with food was all wrong. I used it as a comfort, particularly if I was stressed or tired, or both. I used it as a prop, as a short term boost – especially in the evenings when I was on my own. I then tried to solve the problem by embarking on a hundred different diets – so I quickly became a yo-yo dieter. I was a true victim of the diet industry.

I am not any more. I will never go on a diet again – it is much more fun to instead concentrate on eating the healthiest, most nutritious, most colourful and tasty foods I can find.

A radio interviewer said to me recently: 'Haven't you become a bit of a health freak?' Isn't it strange to be called a health freak when all you are doing is trying to eat healthily? Why should that be freakish? In fact, I do still get those cravings for chocolate or alcohol, as I said.

I am not an exercise junkie. I have just managed, though, to find some forms of exercise which I like, and I stick to them. But you will never get me jogging, or running the marathon – because I just can't bear running! I'm not mad about aerobics, either. And if anyone ever tries to get me into a 'step' class again, I'll throw the ruddy step at them! The trick is to find something you do like. I love my morning session on the trampoline, I am keen on tennis, I love swimming, and I quite enjoy half an hour in the gym. And I have always wanted to have a go on one of those army assault courses – maybe that's an ambition for some time next year!

But a health freak – not me! In fact, I think I will always have to watch myself, to ensure I don't fall back into slovenly ways! Remember the concept of re-tuning? Well, just gently remind yourself of the way you want to lead your life, and how to achieve it. I think I will have to re-read this book every so often. After all, we all have a lot of un-learning to do, a mountain of advertising and hype to learn to ignore on a daily basis – it's a big task, trying to make the healthy choices, when the world is trying to force you into making unhealthy ones.

And, on top of that, you have also got to make sure you are not becoming a diet bore.

There's nothing worse than going out to dinner with someone, and hearing them rattle on endlessly about how awful/enlightened/easy/difficult their diet is. Or, perhaps, they bore you rigid about how you are eating all the wrong things, and how they are the clever ones.

I promise I will never do that. I just wanted to write down an honest account of what happened to me – how I lost all that *Big Brother* weight, and how I discovered that you don't have to go on being a diet victim – you really can break free of all that rubbish, and find a New You. I really do hope that it helps you. I feel so much better, more energetic, and *so much younger* – that I'd love someone else to benefit, too.

I just hope I've got enough of this new energy for my next challenge. Because this New Me is breaking new territory – after nearly twenty five years in print journalism and then TV and radio, I am trying my hand at the theatre! Firstly, I am treading the boards in a panto (the Wicked Witch in Snow White – great chance for a really super dress!) and then who knows?

Maybe I'll go on to Graham Norton's show (even after all those horrible things he said about me during *Big Brother*) and give him some dietary advice – and force him to eat his words!

appendix a

Jason Vale's 21 day kickstart plan

Before embarking on this life-changing programme, it is strongly advised that you read through the entire 21 day and beyond programme. You will discover certain guidelines which will prove essential to your success, together with full explanations of why the programme has been structured the way it has. There are also suggestions for 'eating out during the first 21 days', ideas on how to make lunch and tips on keeping it fresh until lunchtime.

As you are embarking on an entirely new way of eating, it is highly advisable to consult your GP before starting on the 21 day plan. This plan is not recommended whilst you are pregnant, breastfeeding or have an active medical condition.

You should by now be in the right frame of mind to start the plan. If you have any worries or questions – now or at any time during the programme – you can phone 0845 1 30 28 29 or email Anne or Jason at www.thejuicemaster.com.

Day 1 & 2: The Kickstart

The first two days of this programme have been designed to simply 'kickstart' what will turn into a lifelong healthy eating programme. The main purpose of the first two days is to supply your system with nutrition in a liquefied form only, to help aid digestion. Giving your digestive system a break from dealing with cooked and processed food for a couple of days may be extremely beneficial, as some studies have asserted. Dr Roy Walford has written five books on the subject of immunology and ageing, based on his numerous long-term experiments on ageing in animals. He found that simply by resting the digestive systems, a life span could be doubled. Now we're not suggesting for a second that by doing the first two days of this programme once a week for the rest of your life you would live to be one hundred and fifty, but it does illustrate how it may be beneficial to give your system a rest from trying to digest mounds of processed food. This is why the first two days have been designed in the way they have – they are a central component of the programme. So if you really want success it is vital that you follow the first two days to the letter, in order to clear through the built up 'food traffic' in your body. You'll then be ready to reap the huge benefits of the entire 21 day programme *and beyond*. Although these days may appear difficult on paper you will be amazed at just how easy they can be, especially as each 'smoothie meal' has been designed to supply the essential nutrients that your body needs:

- Amino acids (the building blocks for protein)
- Natural Sugars
- Vitamins
- Minerals
- Essential fatty acids
- Water

The smoothies and juices will not supply *all* of these in adequate amounts to hit the government's 'recommended daily intake' guidelines, but please remember that this is only for the first couple of days. Days one and two are *not* meant to be adopted for any longer than the period suggested so please do keep to the programme.

Each smoothie meal provides the six human needs in an easily digestible form. And there is another benefit. Dr Norman Walker, a renowned nutritional and juicing expert in the US, believes that 95% of a vegetable's nutrients remain in its juice when the vegetable is juiced raw. So, because the vegetables are used raw, they generally contain a higher percentage of nutrients than a lot of the processed and cooked foods that you might otherwise consume.

You will notice that about fifteen to twenty minutes after having a smoothie meal you feel surprisingly satisfied, on a physical hunger level. This is due to the fact that your cells have just been fed 'raw' nutrients in the fastest possible way. Although each 'smoothie meal' contains water, we recommend that you drink an additional 2 litres of water daily *throughout* the 21 day programme.

PLEASE NOTE: Please be aware that if you are going from a diet high in refined sugars and processed foods straight into the 21 day programme (as is usually the case) you may well experience some 'withdrawal pangs'. Each smoothie meal will help to combat this by hydrating the system, while also supplying the body with a natural source of sugar, some protein and fat. If you do experience any adverse symptoms such as headaches or weakness, please drink some water and get as much rest as possible. Although your energy levels will increase fairly soon into the 21 day programme, they can dip initially due to the withdrawal of refined sugars and carbohydrates. Please do not panic and certainly do not get deluded into thinking you had more genuine energy before you started. Most people who have refined sugar 'highs' inevitably experience sugar lows afterwards. In their attempt to feel 'balanced' they eat or drink more refined sugars and carbohydrates to 'lift' themselves. What you are doing during this programme is cleansing your system of this refined sugar roller coaster in order to truly balance the body. Happy cleaning!

Days 3 – 5

Now that your system has been free from cooked and heavily processed foods for two days we can incorporate some natural whole foods in the next five days. We are still keeping on the 'nothing but raw' theme, but instead of converting everything into a liquid, it's time that we had something to get our teeth into. The most important part of the first seven days is to lessen the burden on the digestive system; to keep your sugar levels in check and to make sure that nothing passes your lips except 'raw' foods and drinks. This will free up a tremendous amount of nerve energy – which will help to aid weight loss and cleanse the body of waste. Please remember that it is only the first seven days which are 'nothing but natural' days – and it's only the first 5 days which are void of fruit only smoothies and juices.

Days 6 & 7

As I have found that people tend to start the programme on a Monday, and because I know that people's eating habits generally change slightly at the weekends, I have devised days six and seven to fit in with this schedule. The first week of the 21 day programme deliberately leaves out pure fruit smoothies, due to their tendency to raise blood sugar levels too rapidly. However, as it's the weekend, you can enjoy the delicious tastes of these amazing fruit smoothies without causing yourself any problems at all – just so long as you follow my fruit smoothie guidelines (see *recipes*)!

You will notice that I have included some 'live' yoghurt in the smoothies of days six and seven. Although not strictly 'raw' this kind of yoghurt does contain some 'live' friendly bacteria – in other words, it's good for you. You will also see that the main course salad for days six and seven is the same. Don't worry – you *will* see much, much more variety in your meals from day eight and beyond!

Please remember, if you *do* have any feelings of deprivation while on the plan, these feelings will more than likely be mental rather than physical. Any physical 'empty' feelings will usually be 'withdrawal' from processed foods and drinks, instead of any genuine hunger. If in doubt, eat some fruit from the suggested fruit table (see page 245) or some vegetables (any vegetable is fine – but not cooked carrots or white potatoes). Or you could have a delicious veggie juice – whatever you do never go *genuinely* hungry. Remember that one of the most important parts of this life-changing programme is to starve the false hungers (that refined sugar roller coaster) and get into a good healthy eating routine.

Days six and seven are the last two days of the 'kickstart clean'. Remember that it will feel weird – it's probably your first weekend ever where you're eating and drinking nothing but natural foods! – but in the scheme of things it's not hard work. Hold on to your ultimate goal; it only becomes hard if you make it so. Eliminate the mental CANT (Constant And Never-ending Tantrum!) syndrome and there really is no Tantrum or Torture. Happy weekend cleaning!

Days 8 – 21

Please read before continuing

You will no doubt be pleased to hear that the 'cooked food' boycott is now over (hooray!). As your system is a lot cleaner and probably much more balanced than it once was, we can now move on to the next part of the programme. This is where things get a lot, lot easier and where you will really start to enjoy some of the scrummy recipes we have in store…

The programme from here on in couldn't be easier to follow or to understand. You will notice that each day still starts with a fruit or veggie juice or a smoothie. (After the initial 21 day plan the 'flexie breakfast', which incorporates whole food breakfasts, will come into play – but more on that later.) You will also notice that the general theme is a carbohydrate lunch and a protein rich dinner, both combined with high water content, rich in nutrients, salads and steamed veggies.

For most of the initial 21 day plan only one concentrated food is eaten at a time. You are more than welcome, indeed encouraged, to introduce your own recipes during this section – providing you follow 'The Juice Master's Guidelines' (see page 188). Please read these thoroughly before starting the next part of the programme and your future way of living and eating. Remember, the first 7 days were something you were 'on': but from here on in it's a way of life, becoming even more flexible after day 21!

Snacks: Days 8 – 21 and beyond

Now you may be surprised to see this section here. But I'm a realist. And although the meals and juices recommended on the 21 day plan are packed full of energy-giving nutrients and, in my experience, are more than capable of filling you up to the brim, people do tend to snack. I don't recommend it personally, and you should be careful not to let snacking become a regular habit. But sometimes it happens – if you've had a stressful morning, a jumbo workout, a hectic afternoon. As with all food, you should only eat if you are *genuinely* hungry. And rather than reach for that all-too-convenient bag of crisps, or the handy chocolate bar, or the white flour muffin, think about what you are eating and look around. There are plenty of healthy snacks out there which will fill the gap until the next meal without ruining your new routine. Snacks should only be eaten from day eight on the plan and they shouldn't form a regular part of your eating habits. As a guideline, make sure snacks are eaten no less than three hours after a meal and have no more than two snacks a day. Any carbohydrate snacks should be eaten before 6pm.

The idea behind this programme is to make life as easy as possible. One of the biggest excuses people give for not being able to eat healthily is that they don't have the time. But how long does it take to prepare an apple? What about a banana? Or how about a brazil nut? The beauty of Nature is that she has provided us with ready-to-eat snacks which are easy to digest, bursting with nutrients and require no washing up! All we have to do is either grow them or buy them. Our job is actually very easy. Nature has provided literally thousands of these ready made snacks, all bursting with different flavours and all very good for you. Nature's choice is just too long to list and would require a book in itself! However, all you need to do is go down to your local greengrocers or the first aisle of your supermarket and you will see an array of fresh, light, nature-made snacks, such as fresh fruit, nuts, dried fruits and vegetables. All very tasty! See the fruit chart on page 245 for some suggestions of my favourite fruits to snack on.

I am aware, however, that despite the thousands of different fruits, nuts, dried fruits and vegetables on offer from nature's kitchen, sometimes you just want something else. With that in mind I have provided some snack alternatives to fruit and nuts (see page 207 and *recipes*). I would recommend that wherever possible you have a piece of fruit or some nuts as a snack, but these suggestions offer a little more choice if you're in the mood for something different. As a reminder, snacks should only be eaten from day eight and beyond, never during the first week of 'nothing but natural' foods, and never without a genuine hunger for sustenance. You have started this programme because you want to succeed and you will only succeed by understanding and following the guidelines. The best guideline when it comes to snacks is to skip them and let your hunger build – so that you can really appreciate and savour the flavours of your main meals when you have them.

The Juice Master's Guidelines

The 6pm carbohydrate boycott

You may have spotted that at no point during the 21 day plan do you see any evening meals containing 'man-made carbohydrates'. Of course, *all* fruits and vegetables contain carbohydrates, but because they haven't been processed in any way they are not classed as 'man-made carbs'. By 'man-made carbs' I mean foods such as rice, bread, pasta, baked *white* potatoes, chips, and so on. Please note that any 'man-made carbs' which I *do* recommend are always of the 'whole' variety. In other words, they are always as close to the natural grain from which they came as possible. This ensures that they are full of fibre – and will therefore slow down the absorption of sugars into the bloodstream. This prevents an imbalance in sugar levels and also stops a sudden surge of the 'fat producing' hormone insulin being secreted.

In addition to the 'man-made carb' boycott, I have also – just for the rest of the 21 day plan – left out post 6pm fruit smoothies and juices. I would also discourage the eating of lots of fruit in the evening. Although they aren't 'man-made carbs', some fruits can raise sugar levels too rapidly. The guideline is to have any 'man-made carbs' during the day and to have a protein rich meal in the evening. So, if you do decide to make your own meals, make certain you *never* break the '6pm man-made carb curfew': it really is that important to your success.

Eat as many vegetables and have as many veggie juices as you like

It is extremely difficult to overdo vegetables as your body has a natural cut off point. This natural cut off point is often over-ridden by the abundance of high fat, high sugar snacks available. Steamed and stir-fried veggies are a welcome addition to the plan and, although not fully raw, are actually sometimes better in their lightly cooked form. Raw broccoli, for example, is hard for the body to break down and utilise, whereas once steamed the body has a better chance of actually gaining access to the nutrients. Please feel free to have as many vegetables as you like throughout the rest of the programme and beyond. You *can* overdo veggie juices – but it's difficult to do this because of the cut off point. Always use your common sense and try to keep to no more than two pints a day.

Learn 'how' to eat as well as 'what' to eat

What is of vital importance during this stage, and also vital for life-long success, is that you use your blender efficiently. I do not mean the one on your kitchen work surface; I mean the one in your mouth! Your teeth and mouth are designed to be the ultimate blender. It is imperative that you chew your food thoroughly in order to allow for easy assimilation, digestion and elimination. Apart from exercise and what they actually eat, one of the biggest differences between some slim and overweight people is the speed at which they consume their food. In my experience, most overweight people rush their food – whereas virtually all slim people take their time and chew their food thoroughly. When you are always 'on the next forkful', so to speak, and your mouth is already full, you not only miss the pleasure of savouring the full flavours of your food but you also burden the stomach with an unblended mass. It is imperative that you learn 'how to eat' as well as 'what to eat'. This guideline is once again vital to this programme *and beyond*.

The 20 minute rule

As mentioned previously in these guidelines, many people eat far too quickly. Because of this they tend to eat more than they actually need, as it takes time for the body to register that it's had enough. This is another reason why slower eaters tend to eat less – and so remain slim. Please allow yourself to feel a little dissatisfied after your meal. The guideline here is to wait 20 minutes after you've eaten to give your body a chance to feel satisfied. You will find that nine times out of ten, after the 20 minute wait you simply will not be hungry, as you've fed your cells and your insulin levels have dropped.

Do not eat any cooked food three hours before you sleep

In my experience, it takes an average of three hours for cooked food to leave your stomach and progress to the intestinal tract. Raw food, on the other hand, takes an average of just half an hour and has more or less already been pre-digested by the plant. When you sleep your metabolism slows down massively and so digestion of food becomes harder. The body will still digest the food even if you eat one second before you sleep, but the idea of this lifelong programme is to 'free up' as much energy as possible to aid weight-loss and health. With that in mind this guideline, especially for the 21 day kickstart, is very, very important.

Drink your juices on an empty stomach

For ideal results you should make sure that you drink your juices on an empty stomach. This is why I recommend a juice in the morning and as a starter for lunch or dinner.

Keep to the right portion size

Portion size is really significant during the programme. Many people have a tendency to 'Hoover their food', rather than savour the flavours and eat it slowly. A good meal portion, if genuinely physically hungry, is roughly a one inch high dinner plate full. Clearly you should never 'force' food down and, as long as you eat slowly, your body is probably the best judge of how much *you* should be eating. Please also see the portion guidelines set out in the *recipe* section.

Go 'organic' where possible

As mentioned elsewhere in this book, 'organic' really only means anything when you are talking about meat, fish, fruits, vegetables and salads. With that in mind, try to get organic produce for juices and salads wherever possible. I realise that this isn't always a viable option for everyone – but it can make a difference.

If you're unable to buy organic, always remember to thoroughly wash your fruit and vegetables before using them. Remember they are still very good for you!

Tips for storing juices and smoothies

Now, unless you have something called a 'twin-gear low rpm masticating juice extractor' (!) you will find that freshly made fruit and vegetable juices tend to 'oxidise' (that's spoil to you and me) very rapidly. With that in mind, here's a little tip for keeping your juice or smoothie fresher for longer. Simply get a flask (preferably one of those silver looking 'bullet' shaped ones), remove the lid and store in your freezer. Pour your freshly made juice straight into the flask, seal immediately and put it in fridge once you're at work (or wherever). Hey presto, it's good for lunch! This way you can make your lunch juice first thing in the morning, along with your breakfast juice. It also means you only need to clean the juicer once! For better results, add some lemon or lime juice into the mix, to help prevent the oxidation even further.

What juicer and blender?

The two pieces of equipment which are essential to creating 'A New You' are a good juicer and a good blender. Of all the investments you will make in your kitchen these two will be by far the most beneficial. That's why it's important to ensure that you choose the right equipment – it will equip you for your new life ahead.

Firstly, let's look at juicers. There are many different juicers on the market, ranging from £15 to £1000. Remember that just because something costs more, it doesn't necessarily make it better and vice versa: just because something is cheap, it doesn't make it a bargain. In my opinion, most of the machines around the £15-£30 range are pretty useless. They are fiddly, difficult to clean and you have to stop the machine halfway through a job if you are making more than a glassful of juice. I would recommend a machine which is not too expensive to kick off with (you can always upgrade later if you choose), one which has a large pulp container and a larger-than-average feeder shoot. For convenience, look for those juicers which are dishwasher-compatible and also have the capacity to juice up to three pints without stopping. My personal favourite – and one which meets all the criteria above – is The Juice Master Jnr by Moulinex.

As for blenders, as long as you get the 'jug' type and not the hand held versions, most are pretty much the same. All good electrical stores sell good blenders so they are easily available. My pointers here would be to go for those that specifically blend ice as well as fluids, and to opt for a glass jug wherever possible.

If you need any further tips, check out my website www.thejuicemaster.com for help and pointers. You may be interested to know that Anne and I have teamed up with the people at Moulinex to generate an extra special offer to those purchasing The Juice Master Jnr right now. They're giving away copies of The Juice Master's Ultimate Fast Food Book, which explains everything you ever needed to know about juicing and more, free with every juicer purchased. The book alone is usually £8.99, but when you buy the machine at £39.99 it's yours free. To partake of this special offer, phone the offer hotline on 0845 1 30 28 29 or go to www.thejuicemaster.com and click on 'Juicy Diamond Offer'. This offer is set to close July 2004, but do check in case it's been extended. Happy juicing!

Life after the 21 day kickstart plan

A slim, trim and healthy body for life can only be possible by practising a healthy lifestyle most of the time. The human body is quite ingenious and it can indeed handle just about any combination of processed foods or drinks every now and then. The key to health or disease is what you do *most* of the time. If you have processed foods most of the time, eat quickly, eat as a response to emotion and do little or no exercise – then you will suffer the consequences. These can come in the shape of obesity, diabetes, asthma, skin disorders, heart disease, cancer and so on. However, if you eat a diet rich in raw, high water, high nutrient content foods, regularly lift your spirits with fun driven exercise, eat only when you are genuinely hungry and drink those vegetable juices most of the time: then a lifelong slim, trim energy driven body is yours for the taking. You wouldn't expect to go to the gym for four hours once a week and be fit for life – and so you shouldn't think that eating healthily one day a week could make you healthy for life. It's all about the correct ratio.

The 70% – 30% rule

In my opinion, the ideal daily intake for today's world should consist of about 70% 'live' foods and 30% processed. When I talk about 'live' foods I mean foods which are known to have a high concentration of nutrients and are easy for the body to digest, assimilate and eliminate. These include fruits, vegetables, seeds, nuts, salads and fresh juices. Ideally the 70% of 'live' foods should be split into 50% vegetables and 20% fruits. The remaining 30% of your intake should consist of fish, chicken, whole rice, whole bread, whole pasta, noodles, butter, white cheese and so on. The 70% would also include any veggies that have been juiced or steamed, not necessarily consumed raw.

The 6pm carb boycott

The 6pm carb boycott is an extremely good tool: not just for losing the excess pounds but more importantly *keeping* them off; something which 95% of people who go on 'normal' diets fail to do. This is why this tip is included in my post-plan guidelines as well as being prioritised in the 21 day plan itself. By keeping to the 6pm carbohydrate boycott you immediately prevent yourself from slipping back into old ways and habits. In my experience, one of the most common mistakes made by overweight people (not taking into account their exercise routines – or lack of) is to eat lots of carbohydrates at night. In fact, many overweight people skip breakfast, pick at the odd thing during the day and 'binge' on carbohydrates at night. This practice is one of the best ways to *stay* overweight! It doesn't mean that you should *never* have any carbohydrates ever again after 6pm, but I would strongly advise that you stick to this plan 'most of the time' – at least until you are at your ideal weight. You will find that after you have lost the weight and are concentrating on maintaining your shape you can be more flexible. However, even then I would keep to the 6pm carbohydrate boycott as frequently as you can: it really is one of the best tools for staying slim and keeping your energy high. It also stops you having the 'one' biscuit (which always leads to ten!) and avoids picking and having snacks for the sake of it.

Eating out during the 21 day plan

Days 1 and 2 – Eating out during the first two days will be virtually impossible, so please make sure you start this programme at a time when you know you don't have any dinner engagements. Somehow I don't think your friends would be too impressed if you asked for your dinner to be juiced!

Days 3–7 – Eating out during this period is tricky, but not impossible. Ideally you really want to do the 'kickstart seven days' at home, but if your job, family or social life mean that you do need to eat out frequently, then all it needs is a little preparation on your part. Remember that when eating out you are the paying customer – and as such are apparently 'always right'! With that in mind you shouldn't have any difficulty in ordering a main course avocado salad with a light dressing. I appreciate that most salads in restaurants are pretty poor, but you can always say it's 'doctor's orders' and explain that you want a well put together main course salad; i.e. a substantial amount! If out and about during the day it's easy to snack on 'low sugar' fruits (please see fruit chart on page 245 for some examples).

Days 8–21 – Eating out after the initial seven day 'kickstart' couldn't be easier. There probably isn't a restaurant in the world you can't eat at during the rest of the 21 days. That's what's so excellent about this programme once we're past the first seven days – you are free to tuck into good food! The only 'rule' for days 8–21 is that you keep to the 6pm carbohydrate boycott. This is easy to do in any restaurant. All you need to do is order whatever fish or chicken dish they have, and combine it with a salad and/or veggies. Soups are OK to have – but no bread with them. If you're out in a restaurant for lunch you can have anything which takes your fancy! Remember to have plenty of salad or vegetables with your meal, and make sure it doesn't include any white flour. Other than that, just tuck in; remembering to eat slowly and not to leave feeling 'stuffed'.

Drinking while on the 21 day plan

Most people are fine with the majority of the first 21 days, but many say, 'WHAT ABOUT MY TEA AND COFFEE?!' Please remember that the idea behind these first 21 days is to change your eating and drinking habits. Try drinking peppermint, camomile, or lemon tea – all these are caffeine free. You can have a small spoonful of manuka active honey in the drinks to sweeten them, if necessary. One of the most cleansing hot drinks – and one which you will soon get into the habit of having – is some hot water with a couple of slices of lemon and lime: it sounds weird but don't knock it until you've tried it!

Alcohol!

Over 90% of the UK drinks alcohol on a fairly regular basis. Most will tell you they don't have a problem and that they could stop whenever they like. Well, if that really is the case then not drinking for 21 days should be a piece of cake. However, the reality is very different. Although people say they don't have a problem, the majority believe they couldn't enjoy or cope with their lives without it. I would like you to give yourself the freedom of having a non-drink, just for 21 days as part of this programme. After that a couple of glasses of red or white wine or the odd beer is not going to affect your success. The problem is that most people don't seem to be able to have 'just the one' – and before they know it have gone on to two or three or four or floor! Alcohol addiction is another subject entirely and clearly I cannot go into it here in any depth. If you do feel you have a problem, please go to www.thejuicemaster.com and click on 'Stop Drinking 4 Life'.

Best takeaway

The following advice is for *after* the first 21 days. The choice of takeaways out there is pretty poor to say the least. However, I'm a realist and there's no question that there will be times when you can't be bothered to prepare a meal and fancy something super quick. The best takeaway for the healthy lifestyle is a Chinese. The only problem here is that restaurants tend to put loads of Mono Sodium Glutamate (MSG) in the food. This is a flavouring which, in short, just isn't good for your health. If you say that you're allergic to MSG, however, they will leave it out. This also means that you will get your food fresh, as they will almost certainly have to make up some without the flavouring. Now I know that the rice you get is not 'whole rice' and is an undisputed 'man-made carb' – but takeaways are something you won't be doing most of the time, so it's fine on these rare occasions. Boiled rice would be your best bet. You can also get plenty of mixed vegetables in a Chinese takeaway and some lean meats, prawns and noodles. Indian is another good option as it can often be 'light' and getting veggies shouldn't be difficult. The worst of the bunch – and in my mind these premises should never be entered at all! – are the big name fast food 'joints': I think you know who they are.

Additions after the 21 days

As you have seen, the 21 day programme initiates you into some life-changing practices and is a way of life for life. As the 21 day programme should only be followed within that allotted time span, however, please feel free to introduce some other foods, such as more dairy products, after the 21 days, and please remember to be flexible. There will be times in your future life when you won't be able to get fresh produce or a good piece of organic fish with steamed veggies – and times when you want something more for breakfast than just juice. If so, please understand that the body can deal with small amounts of anything – it's what you do *most* of the time that counts. So if you want some muesli and rye toast in the morning, or some boiled eggs – tuck in! When introducing dairy, I would advise organic white cheeses (like Cheshire) and semi-skimmed milk. You are welcome to re-introduce red meat to your diet if you wish, although personally I am not a fan. If you do please make sure you get a good cut from a good source and avoid any meats that are combined or encased in things like pigs' intestines (sausages for example!). Happy eating!

What about on holiday?

Many people will say it's hard to be healthy on holiday, but once again it's just not true. Often the weather is better and fruits are available aplenty. Most restaurants serve wonderful fresh fish and have a good supply of vegetables. People only think it's hard because they always tend to 'binge' whilst away. Holidays are a great time to eat well, sleep well, take in some good air and do plenty of exercise. Use them to do just that!

Please note that even if you've been on this programme and way of thinking for months, old patterns can come forward. For example, if you go on holiday and it's your first holiday eating this way, then it's perfectly natural for you to 'think' the old way. This doesn't mean that you are genuinely craving the other stuff, it's just an old image from your brain coming forward. As long as you see it for what it is you will learn to enjoy your holiday without having to binge.

Health rules for life!

1. No white flour whatsoever!
2. 70% 'live' foods *daily*.
3. Get veggie juiced every day!
4. Processed and refined foods in emergencies and 'when in Rome' moments only.
5. 6pm carb boycott.
6. Eat only when genuinely hungry.
7. Leave at least three hours after main meals before eating anything.
8. Have a 'Natural Day' one day every week – 'live' foods only all day!
9. Two lots of 20 minute stints of 'exercise till you sweat' every day.
10. 6–8 hours of sleep/rest daily.
11. Never eat any cooked food three hours before you sleep.
12. Always have something exciting to look forward to.

appendix b

21 day kickstart: the meal plan

Days 1 & 2 *The Kickstart*

NOTE – Drink either a glass or mug of cold water with slices of fresh lemon and lime half an hour before you go to bed. You may also replace the cold water in the morning for a mug of hot water with lemon and lime.

Day 1

Morning	Large glass of water with slice of lemon/lime
	The Juice Master's Wake Up Smoothie
Lunch	The Juice Master's Super Cleaner
Dinner	The Juice Master's Master Juice

Anne's Tip of the Day

Plan loads of things to do to keep you busy for the next two days. Don't make the mistake of thinking you won't have energy – you will have lots! Keep away from the kitchen as much as possible. Keep a water bottle with you at all times so that you drink, drink, drink and don't let yourself get bored.

Day 2

Morning	Large glass of water with slice of lemon/lime
	The Juice Master's Wake Up Smoothie
Lunch	The Juice Master's Lunch Tonic
Dinner	The Juice Master's Master Smoothie

Anne's Tip of the Day

Buy a box of assorted herbal teas, and try a different flavour every time you feel like a hot drink. I have a reflex action where every time I go into the kitchen, I click the kettle on! If you have the same need to have a regular cuppa, then make yourself a herbal tea – and get the hell out of the kitchen! Go to bed early tonight with a good book or watch a movie in bed – or better still, take your partner with you...

Days 3 – 21

Please note: from now on if you feel *genuinely* hungry at any point you are free to have as many vegetable juices as you like, as many raw vegetables and as many low sugar fruits as your body desires (see fruit guide page 245). Please be careful to eat only if genuinely hungry and not as a response to emotion. Even good foods can cause problems if you are eating them when your body is not really hungry.

Day 3

Morning	Large glass of water with slice of lemon/lime
	The Juice Master's Wide Awake Smoothie
Lunch	Jasey's Apple, Pear, Cinnamon and Raisin Salad
Dinner	The Juice Master's Flusher
	Followed by Jasey's Three Leaf Salad

Anne's Tip of the Day

Savour every mouthful of smoothie and salad – you've earned it! By slowly relishing every gram of food or drink, you will learn to appreciate the taste of good, whole food and you will also learn the great habit of eating slowly – something we rarely do nowadays.

Day 4

Morning	Large glass of water with slice of lemon/lime
	The Juice Master's Wake Up Smoothie
Lunch	Jasey's Over The Moon Salad

Dinner	The Juice Master's Fire Starter
	Followed by Jasey's Hey Pesto Salad

Anne's Tip of the Day

When I did the 21 day plan, by this time I was feeling just a little sick, and I couldn't understand why, since I was possibly the healthiest I had ever been. It's a common reaction, apparently, to fasting (which is almost what you have done for the past three days). That's why you will find the ginger in your Fire Starter juice very handy, as ginger will stop any feelings of nausea. It's also thought that ginger boosts calorie burning!

Day 5

Morning	Large glass of water with slice of lemon/lime
	The Juice Master's Green, Mean, Wake Up Machine
Lunch	Melon Magic
Dinner	Jasey's Avocado and Cos Lettuce Wrap, with Veggie Juice

Anne's Tip of the Day

By now you will probably be starting to feel the effects of detoxing. At about this time, I noticed my skin was getting spotty. Fear not! It will improve again – the body is cleaning itself out. Brace yourself for a whole melon for lunch! It sounds extravagant, and yet costs less than a mug of Pot Noodles and a chocolate bar – and is far more nutritious. We have come to think of fruit as a luxury item and of processed, expensive junk as regular food. Remember that every mouthful of what you are eating now is 100% goodness. And avocado for supper? I was surprised this was included since most 'diets' rule out avocados. It's very good for you, though, with vital nutrients, and healthy oils.

Day 6

Breakfast	Large glass of water with slice of lemon/lime
	The Juice Master's Let's Get Fruity
Lunch	The Juice Master's Master Juice
Dinner	The Juice Master's Flusher
	Followed by The Juice Master's Master Salad

Anne's Tip of the Day

Remember to keep drinking water – keep that bottle with you! And retune your mind by listening again and again to your retuning CD, or re-reading your favourite chapters from the book. You may think you know all the facts, but going over them again and again will help your subconscious mind make the right decisions. I cannot emphasise how important this is.

Day 7

Breakfast	Large glass of water with slice of lemon/lime
	The Juice Master's Wakey Wakey
Lunch	Jasey's Beautiful Fruit 'n' Nut Salad
Dinner	The Juice Master's Make A Start
	Followed by The Juice Master's Master Salad

Anne's Tip of the Day

This is the last day of 'no protein', so don't worry or lose heart if you are feeling hungry. You have done brilliantly well! But remember this is not a diet, it's a truly healthy way of living. Your body is a Ferrari, and you've just got rid of all the old, mucky oil and replaced it with the best, clean, refined oil so that the engine will run like a dream.

Day 8

Morning	Large glass of water with slice of lemon/lime
	The Juice Master's Morning Glory
Lunch	JM's Take the Edge Off
Dinner	The Juice Master's Heavenly Trout

Anne's Tip of the Day

I was never a great fish lover – but by the time you get to this day, you will relish every mouthful with a new spirit! Eat it slowly though, and concentrate on the individual tastes. You are not only learning to eat healthier food, you are re-learning how to eat – slowly and surely does it!

Day 9

Morning	Large glass of water with slice of lemon/lime
	The Juice Master's Wide Awake Juice
Lunch	JM's Whole Grain Super Sandwich
Dinner	The Juice Master's 'Monk'ey Magic with a Broccoli Kicker

Anne's Tip of the Day

Sometimes it can be hard making every day's different juice: you have to have a kitchen load of fruit and veggies (my kitchen counters always look like a greengrocer's!) and yet it all goes so quickly! So if you have found a favourite morning juice by now, then stick to making that. During these 21 days, however, try to follow Jason's recipes for lunch and dinner, as they are carefully worked out to give you maximum nutrition.

Day 10

Morning	Large glass of water with slice of lemon/lime
	The Juice Master's Morning Gorgeous
Lunch	Jasey's Hummus Cool Dipper
Dinner	The Juice Master's Steamed Cuisine

Anne's Tip of the Day

Yes – you can have hummus! This is where I started to realise that this eating plan is not about denial and giving up all the things you find tasty. If it is healthy, made with the best, fresh ingredients, then you can have it. I always used to eat hummus with breadsticks or sliced baguette. Nowadays, though, I wouldn't want to mess up the taste with unwanted white, refined carbohydrate. Eaten with fresh veggies instead, the whole meal becomes 100% healthy.

Day 11

Morning	Large glass of water with slice of lemon/lime
	The Juice Master's Wake Up Smoothie
Lunch	The Juice Master's Master Muesli
Dinner	Jasey's Sultry Salmon with Mango and Asparagus Kicker

Anne's Tip of the Day

I remember Day 11 very well, as this was the first day that I weighed myself – and I had lost eleven pounds! I was so thrilled, I took the family out to supper to celebrate. The kids had pizza, but I had a large plate of smoked salmon and a green salad and felt very proud of myself. You see, you can even go out to dinner on this 21 day plan! (Though please be careful in your menu choices!)

Day 12

Morning	Large glass of water with slice of lemon/lime
	The Juice Master's Minty Magic
Lunch	Caesar Salad
Dinner	Jasey's Tuna Salad with Fresh Pesto and Pineapple

Anne's Tip of the Day

Today you're eating the two meals which have become my staple diet nowadays: the Caesar salad and the tuna salad. The Caesar is so incredibly useful, because most restaurants will serve it and it also comes instant from many high street supermarkets and delis so, if you are stuck for something to eat and you need it quick – hey presto! Even if you don't think you are a great salad person, do stick with them, because I promise you – it's an acquired taste and you will learn to love them!

Day 13

Morning	Large glass of water with slice of lemon/lime
	The Juice Master's Power Smoothie
Lunch	Jasey's Green Power Toasted Wholegrain Sandwich
Dinner	Jasey's Funky Chicken with Buttered Broccoli and Courgettes

Anne's Tip of the Day

You are now more than halfway through the 21 day plan – so you will be feeling the difference. By now, I found it slightly easier going to bed still feeling hungry, because I knew I felt so much better in the mornings. Just remind yourself that for almost a fortnight now you have been fuelling your engine with only the very best food. Those early days of 'detoxing' are over – and your skin will be starting to brighten up again too. Don't go back to your old ways now – keep pressing on!

Day 14

Morning	Large glass of water with slice of lemon/lime
	The Juice Master's Fruity Weekender
Lunch	The Juice Master's Hot 'n' Fishy Snack Attack
Dinner	The Juice Master's Flusher
	Followed by Jasey's Cod 'n' Chips

Anne's Tip of the Day

Fish and chips! Now there's something to look forward to – and another lesson in healthy eating as well. You don't have to give up the things you love; just find healthy ways of eating them. For example, I love tuna pasta bake (tuna with pasta and a mushroom sauce, baked in the oven with breadcrumbs on top). Nowadays I do the same dish but with all-wholemeal ingredients. The kids didn't take to brown, wholemeal pasta at first so I introduced it gradually… and now they love it!

Day 15

Morning	Large glass of water with slice of lemon/lime
	The Juice Master's Morning Lift
Lunch	The Juice Master's Master Smoothie
Dinner	Jasey's Quick 'n' Easy Tuna, Mayo Salad

Anne's Tip of the Day

You are doing brilliantly – but a word of warning. Tell too many friends what you are doing and you may get a negative reaction. Watch out for jealousy (because you are at last succeeding in your battle of the bulge) or for those friends and relatives who like to talk you into eating more 'because it won't do you any harm' or 'you don't want to get too thin'! Others will want to get their opinions in, and will tell you to try their diet, or pooh-pooh what you are doing. Just tell them 'it's working for me' and stick at it.

Day 16

Morning	Large glass of water with slice of lemon/lime
	The Juice Master's Dysun
Lunch	Jasey's Lord Sandwich
Dinner	Jasey's Stir Fried Fish and Veggie Special

Anne's Tip of the Day

I remember after dinnertime on this day, I stayed up late and at midnight, I cooked myself another veggie stir-fry all over again and ate it while watching a late night movie. I felt so guilty and upset that I had done so well for so long, and then cocked it all up on Day 16. In the olden days of dieting, that would have been enough to convince me to give up. But no – if you waver at all, if you succumb to the temptations of a chocolate bar or a packet of crisps, just shrug your shoulders and get on with the next day as if it never happened. Do not allow anything to stop the train you're on – keep moving forwards, never back.

Day 17

Morning	Large glass of water with slice of lemon/lime
	The Juice Master's Green, Mean, Wake Up Machine
Lunch	Jasey's Clear Skin Flusher
	Followed 15 minutes later by Stuffed Pepper Supreme with Pesto
Dinner	Jasey's Lip Licking Lemon Chicken (if veggie replace with quorn fillet)

Anne's Tip of the Day

Let me remind you at this stage to keep 'retuning' – by reading the book over and over again, or listening to your retuning CD. This 21 day plan is not just a diet, it is about learning a new philosophy about food – *and* fitness. Are you doing something active every day? Ten minutes brisk walking down the road, a game of tennis or an outing to the swimming pool? Exercise must become as much of a habit as your new-style eating. Build it in somehow!

Day 18

Morning Large glass of water with slice of lemon/lime
The Juice Master's Wide Awake Smoothie

Lunch The Juice Master's Master Salad *(light version)*

Dinner Jasey's Honey-glazed Salmon, Papaya and Rocket Salad

Anne's Tip of the Day

If you are still not a great water drinker, then try flavouring it. I used to buy bottles of flavoured water, until I realised that they don't use fruit juices to flavour it, they use sugar or a chemical sugar substitute. Very healthy, I don't think! So I started pouring the tiniest amount of orange or pineapple juice (and I do mean only about a millimetre at the bottom of the glass) into water. At first, it tastes odd, but (the old phrase) you do get used to it! It is very important to get into the water habit – so persevere.

Day 19

Morning Large glass of water with slice of lemon/lime
The Juice Master's Morning Gorgeous

Lunch The Iron Lady
Followed by Jasey's Tuna Mayo and Rye Bread Snack Attack

Dinner Jasey's Fish Kebabs with Pineapple and Steamed Veggies

Anne's Tip of the Day

You have now gone 19 days without eating a man-made carbohydrate after 6pm – and to be honest, if you could stick to that habit for the rest of your life, it would be the single best way to ensure that you slowly but surely lose weight. It hasn't been so hard, has it? I have made this a new habit – and I now think that the single biggest thing that caused my weight problem was my addiction to late night carbs! I used to eat a mountain of pasta or rice in the evenings. I can honestly say that I have kicked my addiction, but if I ever fancy a sarnie or a pasta or rice dish in the evenings now, I promise myself that I'll have it the next day – just before 6pm.

Day 20

Morning	Large glass of water with slice of lemon/lime
	The Juice Master's Morning Weekend Lift
Lunch	Jasey's Quick 'n' Easy Hot Pittas and Dip
Dinner	Jasey's Juicy Red Starter
	Followed by Hot 'n' Cold Veggie Delight

Anne's Tip of the Day

Remember to eat everything very slowly – including your morning juice or smoothie. Experts reckon that it takes your brain 20 minutes to register that your stomach is full. (Odd that, considering that if someone punches you in the stomach, your brain registers it straight away!) Whether or not this conjecture is true, it does seem to work. If you still feel a little hungry after a meal, go off and do something distracting for 20 minutes and usually, the hunger pangs will disappear without you noticing. Anyhow, the slower you eat, the more you will aid the digestive system and the better eating habits you will build up. Too many people stuff their food nowadays, giving them time only to stuff some more. Learn to 'eat like a fairy', as my mum would say!

Day 21

Morning	Large glass of water with slice of lemon/lime
	The Juice Master's Power Smoothie
Lunch	The Juice Master's Lunch Tonic
	Followed by Pitta Bread Salad
Dinner	Fresh Tuna with Cracked Pepper and Coriander with Rocket Salad

Anne's Tip of the Day

By now you'll be waking up craving your morning juice – it is amazing how quickly you get used to new habits. In fact, scientists reckon 21 days is the minimum time in which the average human can 'unlearn' a habit and learn a new one. Could be why we called this the 21 day plan! The idea was to keep you energised, with maximum nutrition yet low calories, and to show you how interesting healthy eating can be. Was even one of those meals boring?!

Tomorrow is the beginning of a new you. Read, re-read and read again those 'Health Rules For Life' – that way you can eat anything you like, because you know how good it is *and* you understand why. Good luck for the future – and remember, if you succeed in your aim just 51% of the time, you are winning. If you can do better than that, it will show in your body shape and your whole attitude to life.

Snack suggestions

Days 8–21 and beyond only

Please note: Make sure these snacks are eaten no less than three hours after a meal; no more than two snacks a day. Any carbohydrate snacks must be eaten before 6pm.

Avocado and Sardines

JM's Snack Attack

JM's Small Cucumber Dipper

JM's Wholemeal Pitta Snack

JM's Sun-dried Tomatoes and Olives

Tinned Fish Snack

Organic Rye Crackers

Oat Cakes

Soups

Organic Boiled Eggs

Juicy Snack

Dried Fruits and Nuts

Organic Date and Apricot Slices

The Best Snack of All

appendix c

recipes for success!

Juices and Smoothies

Remember to drink the juices and smoothies very slowly and treat them like a meal. Fruits and vegetables need to be washed but should be left unpeeled except if stated otherwise. Chop fruits and vegetables as necessary to feed into the juicer.

The Juice Master's Wake Up Smoothie

Serves 2

Ingredients:

1 stick celery	½ ripe avocado, flesh only
½ cucumber	¼ lime, peeled
4 apples	small handful of ice
½ pineapple, peeled	

Instructions:

Juice the cucumber, celery, pineapple, lime and 3 of the apples. Place the avocado and the remaining apple into a blender together with the juice mixture and ice. Blend for 45 seconds.

The Juice Master's Super Cleaner

Serves 1

Ingredients:

4 carrots   1 inch fresh ginger

4 apples

Instructions:

Juice all the ingredients together.

The Juice Master's Master Juice

Serves 1–2

Ingredients:

2 sticks celery   2 cups spinach

½ small cucumber   ½ small pineapple, peeled

3 apples   1 ripe avocado, flesh only

1 inch fresh ginger   small handful of ice

Instructions:

Juice the pineapple, celery, apples, cucumber, ginger, and spinach. Place the avocado into blender along with ice and the juice mixture. Blend for 45 seconds.

The Juice Master's Lunch Tonic

Serves 1–2

Ingredients:

3 apples   1 inch fresh ginger

¼ turnip   small handful of ice

2 carrots   pinch of cinnamon

Instructions:

Juice all the ingredients, add ice and stir in the pinch of cinnamon.

The Juice Master's Master Smoothie

Serves 2

Ingredients:

2 sticks celery	½ yellow pepper
4 apples	½ orange pepper
4 carrots	¼ lime, peeled
1 cup spinach	1 ripe avocado, flesh only
1 cup broccoli	small handful of ice

Instructions:

Juice 3 of the apples, the celery, carrots, spinach, broccoli, peppers and lime. Place the avocado in a blender together with the juice mixture and add ice. Blend for one minute.

The Juice Master's Wide Awake Smoothie

Serves 1–2

Ingredients:

4 carrots	¼ lime, peeled
3 apples	small handful of ice
½ pineapple, peeled	

Instructions:

Juice the carrots, half of the apples, pineapple and lime. Put the remaining apples into the blender, add juice mixture and ice. Blend for one minute.

The Juice Master's Flusher

Serves 1

Ingredients:

½ cucumber   1 stick celery

2 apples   ¼ lime, peeled

Instructions:

Juice all the ingredients together. Add ice before serving.

The Juice Master's Fire Starter

Serves 1

Ingredients:

1 inch fresh ginger   3 apples

½ red pepper

Instructions:

Juice all the ingredient together. Add ice before serving.

The Juice Master's Green, Mean, Wake Up Machine

Serves 1–2

Ingredients:

½ cucumber   6 green apples

1 stick celery   ¼ lime, peeled

1 cup spinach   ½ inch fresh ginger

Instructions:

Juice all the ingredients together. Add ice before serving.

The Juice Master's Let's Get Fruity

Serves 2–3

Ingredients:

1 banana, peeled

Small handful of blueberries

½ small mango, flesh only

¼ pineapple, peeled

4 oranges, peeled

½ cup 'live' yogurt (preferably goat's)

10 almonds

small handful of ice

Instructions:

Juice the pineapple and oranges. Place the mango, banana, blueberries, yogurt, nuts into blender with the juice mixture and ice. Blend for 45 seconds.

Please Note. If allergic to nuts please simply leave out of recipe.

The Juice Master's Wakey Wakey

Serves 1–2

Ingredients:

½ grapefruit, peeled

½ pineapple, peeled

1 passion fruit, flesh only

1 cup 'live' yogurt (preferably
   goat's)

4 Brazil nuts

2 kiwi fruit, peeled

small handful of ice

Instructions:

Juice the grapefruit and pineapple. Place nuts, yogurt, passion fruit and kiwi fruit in the blender together with the juice mixture and ice. Blend for one minute.

Please note: Drink slowly! If too sharp for your tastes, use whole pineapple and omit grapefruit.

The Juice Master's Make A Start

Serves 1

Ingredients:

¼ raw beetroot

¼ cup fennel

1 cup broccoli

2 carrots

4 apples

1 cup spinach

small handful of ice

Instructions:

Juice all the ingredients together. Add ice before serving.

The Juice Master's Morning Glory

Serves 2

Ingredients:

½ medium pineapple, peeled

1 cup fresh or frozen
  blueberries

½ cup fresh or frozen
  blackberries

½ banana, peeled

½ cup 'live' yogurt (preferably goat's)

pinch of cinnamon

small handful of ice

Instructions:

Juice the pineapple. Place berries, banana and yogurt in a blender together with pineapple juice, cinnamon and ice. Blend for one minute.

The Juice Master's Wide Awake Juice

Serves 1–2

Ingredients:

1 pineapple, peeled

8 fresh or frozen strawberries

¼ pink grapefruit, peeled

handful of ice

Instructions:

Juice the pineapple and grapefruit. Place strawberries, juice mixture and ice in a blender. Blend for 45 seconds.

The Juice Master's Morning Gorgeous

Serves 1

Ingredients:

¼ cucumber

2 sticks celery

3 apples

¼ pineapple, peeled

¼ lime, peeled

Instructions:

Juice the pineapple and lime. Place the cucumber, celery and apples in a blender together with juice mixture and ice. Blend for 1 minute.

The Juice Master's Minty Magic

Serves 1

Ingredients:

¼ pineapple, peeled

¼ cucumber

1 stick celery

2 apples

eggcup raw beetroot

Fresh mint for garnish

Instructions:

Juice the ingredients together. Add ice and sprinkle fresh mint on top before serving.

The Juice Master's Power Smoothie

Serves 1–2

Ingredients:

1 banana, peeled

1 cup 'live' yogurt

large pinch of cinnamon

4 fresh apricots, cored

1 peach

small handful of ice

Instructions:

Place all of the ingredients into a blender together with half of the cinnamon. Blend for 45 seconds. Sprinkle with remaining cinnamon before serving.

The Juice Master's Fruity Weekender

Serves 1

Ingredients:

Large handful fresh berries
    (any kind)

½ banana, peeled

1 conference pear

½ pineapple, peeled

small handful of ice

Instructions:

Juice the pineapple and pear. Place the banana and berries in a blender, together with the juice mixture and ice. Blend for 45 seconds.

The Juice Master's Morning Lift

Serves 1

Ingredients:

5 apples	1 cup spinach
1 inch fresh ginger	pinch nutmeg
¼ lime, peeled	small handful of ice
small handful fennel	

Instructions:

Juice all the fruits and vegetables together. Add ice and nutmeg before serving.

The Juice Master's Dysun

Serves 2

Ingredients:

3 apples	¼ medium cucumber
3 carrots	2 cups spinach
1 palm-sized raw beetroot	small handful of ice
2 sticks celery	

Instructions:

Juice all the ingredients together. Add ice before serving.

Jasey's Clear Skin Flusher

Serves 1

Ingredients:

½ cucumber	½ inch of fresh ginger

1 stick celery   small handful of ice

2 large apples

Instructions:

Juice all the ingredients together. Add ice before serving.

The Iron Lady

Serves 1

Ingredients:

3 apples   1 cup spinach

3 carrots   small handful of ice

½ cup broccoli

Instructions:

Juice all the ingredients together. Add ice before serving.

The Juice Master's Morning Weekend Lift

Serves 1

Ingredients:

½ banana, peeled   ½ small ripe mango, flesh only

1 passion fruit, flesh only   cupful of ice

4 oranges, peeled

Instructions:

Juice the oranges. Place passion fruit, banana and mango in a blender together with the orange juice and ice. Blend for 45 seconds.

Jasey's Juicy Red Starter

Serves 1

Ingredients:

1 stick celery	3 apples
¼ cucumber	small handful of fennel
½ small red beetroot	small handful of ice

Instructions:

Juice all the ingredients together. Add ice before serving.

Lunches and Dinners

For the sake of this programme our guidelines for evening protein meals are 8–12 ounces of white meat or fish, combined with at least 4 cups of various colours of vegetables and lunch guideline is 6–8 ounces of carbohydrate (whole grain rice, whole pasta, baked potato etc.). Bread guideline is no more than 2 thin slices of wholemeal or rye bread combined with large salad and/or 2–4 cups of vegetables.

Apple, Pear, Cinnamon and Raisin Salad

Serves 1

Ingredients:

2 apples, diced	pinch of cinnamon
1 conference pear, diced	handful of raisins.

Instructions:

Place the apples and pear into bowl. Add raisins and sprinkle cinnamon on top.

Jasey's Three Leaf Salad

Serves 2

Ingredients:

2 cups spinach

1 cup watercress

1 cup Romaine lettuce

¼ cucumber, chopped

3 spring onion bulbs, chopped

1 orange pepper, chopped

¼ cup white cabbage, grated

¼ cup red cabbage, grated

½ celery stick, chopped

4 'unsulphured' dried apricots

½ lemon

½ lime

eggcupful cold pressed virgin olive oil

Instructions:

Place spinach, watercress and Romaine lettuce into small salad bowl. Add cucumber, orange pepper and spring onion on top of the three leaves. Add white and red cabbages, celery and apricots. Squeeze the juice from both the lemon and lime over the salad along with olive oil. Toss salad and serve immediately.

Jasey's Over The Moon Salad

Serves 2

Ingredients:

2 cups rocket leaves

1 cup spinach

¼ cup walnuts

½ red pepper, diced

1 apple

small handful of raisins

½ lemon

½ lime

eggcupful cold pressed virgin olive oil

Instructions:

Tear the rocket and spinach leaves into salad bowl. Add walnuts, diced pepper, apple and raisins. Squeeze the juice from the lemon and lime over the salad, add olive oil. Toss salad and serve immediately.

Jasey's Hey Pesto Salad

Serves 1

Ingredients:

Salad

1 cup watercress

1 beef tomato, sliced thickly

2 large ripe avocados, flesh only,
   cut into quarters

Pesto

⅓ cup fresh basil,
   finely chopped

handful of pine nuts

eggcupful cold pressed virgin olive oil

1 clove garlic

1 lemon

Instructions:

Place watercress on top of the sliced tomato on a plate. Add avocados.

   Make the pesto with basil leaves, pine nuts, olive oil and garlic by pounding in a pestle and mortar. If you don't have a pestle and mortar simply add everything into a cup and mix. Add pesto to the salad together with the juice from the lemon.

Melon Magic

Serves 2 (depending on size of melon)

Ingredients:

1 whole melon (any except
   watermelon), flesh only,
   chopped

Pinch of cinnamon powder

Instructions:

Place flesh of melon in a bowl, add cinnamon and serve.

Jasey's Avocado And Cos Lettuce Wrap, with Veggie Juice

Serves 1

Ingredients:

2 ripe avocados, flesh only

1 yellow pepper, diced

1 orange pepper, diced

¼ small red onion, diced

1 cup spinach

1 lemon

2 large organic Cos lettuce leaves

Juice

4 carrots

2 apples

¼ cucumber

Instructions:

Place avocados into a bowl and add peppers, red onion and spinach. Add juice from half the lemon, mix ingredients together and scoop on to the lettuce leaves. Fold over to make a wrap.

Juice the remaining lemon along with carrots, apples and cucumber.

The Juice Master's Master Salad

Serves 2–3

Ingredients:

2 cups spinach leaves

2 cups rocket leaves

½ cup watercress

⅛ cup red cabbage, grated

½ carrot, grated

¼ small cucumber, diced

¼ cup broccoli

1 whole bell pepper (any colour), diced

6 black olives

eggcupful cold pressed virgin olive oil

balsamic vinegar

1 lemon

1 lime

2 medium ripe avocados, flesh only, diced into large chunks

Instructions:

Place spinach, rocket and watercress leaves on plate or small salad bowl. Add red cabbage, carrot, broccoli, cucumber, pepper and black olives on top of salad leaves. Add olive oil, balsamic vinegar and juice from half of the lemon and lime on top of the salad. Toss together. Place avocado on top and squeeze the juice from the remaining lemon and lime on to the avocados.

The Juice Master's Master Salad – *Light Version*

Serves 1–2

Ingredients:

1 cup spinach leaves

1 cup rocket leaves

½ cup watercress

¼ small cucumber, diced

⅛ cup red cabbage, grated

½ carrot, grated

¼ cup broccoli

½ bell pepper (any colour), diced

4 black olives

eggcupful cold pressed virgin olive oil

balsamic vinegar

1 lemon

1 lime

1 medium ripe avocado, flesh only, diced into large chunks

Instructions:

Place spinach, rocket and watercress leaves on a plate, or in a small salad bowl. Add red cabbage, carrot, cucumber, broccoli, pepper, and black olives on top of the salad leaves. Add olive oil and balsamic vinegar and juice from half of the lemon and lime on top. Toss together. Place avocado on top and squeeze the juice from the remaining lemon and lime on to the avocado.

Jasey's Beautiful Fruit 'n' Nut Salad

Serves 1-2

Ingredients:

1 mango, flesh only, chopped

1 kiwi fruit, peeled, chopped

2 apples, chopped

1 Conference pear, chopped

6 almonds, soaked in water overnight

handful of sesame seeds

small handful of raisins.

Instructions:

Place mango, kiwi, apples and pear in a bowl. Sprinkle the almonds, sesame seeds and raisins over the top.

JM's Take The Edge Off

Serves 1

Ingredients:

2 slices rye bread, toasted

1½ ripe avocado, flesh only

1 lemon

2 x 95g can boneless sardines
in sunflower oil, drained

Instructions:

Spread the toasted rye bread with avocado flesh, add sardines on top and serve with a squeeze of lemon juice over the top.

Please note: if vegetarian simply leave sardines and add more avocado.

The Juice Master's Heavenly Trout

Serves 2

Ingredients:

2 whole trout, cleaned

balsamic vinegar

extra virgin olive oil

2 lemons

2 cloves garlic, crushed

½ red pepper, chopped

½ orange pepper, chopped

½ yellow pepper, chopped

1 red onion, chopped finely

some capers

16 black pitted olives

large handful organic broccoli

small handful organic mangetout

Instructions:

Place trout on some foil, brush over with some virgin olive oil. Add some balsamic vinegar and squeeze some lemon juice on to foil. Put crushed garlic into the inside of trout. Stuff a handful of red, orange and yellow peppers together with red onion inside each piece of fish along with 4 olives and a few capers. Squeeze some lemon juice inside fish. Put remaining peppers on the outside of fish, squeeze some more lemon juice and crunch the foil together on top like a Cornish pasty to seal each piece of fish.

Place stuffed trout on a baking tray and bake in preheated hot oven – gas mark no. 7 (220°C or 450°F) for 20 minutes.

Steam the broccoli and mangetout for about 5–7 minutes.

Take fish out, place on warmed plate and add veggies. Place the remaining olives and capers on the cooked fish. Add lemon juice, balsamic vinegar and olive oil over the fish. Serve with a large wine glass full of cool water with slice of lemon.

JM's Whole Grain Super Sandwich

Serves 1

Ingredients:

small amount of mayonnaise   1 cup of alfalfa sprouts

2 slices of wholemeal/grain
  bread

4 slices cucumber

½ ripe avocado, flesh only

½ lemon

Instructions:

Spread a thin layer of mayonnaise on to both slices of bread together with the avocado flesh. On one slice of the bread, add the cucumber and alfalfa sprouts on top, add juice from the lemon, top with the other slice of bread. Cut in half and serve.

The Juice Master's 'Monk'ey Magic with a Broccoli Kicker

Serves 2

Ingredients:

Two 8oz pieces Monkfish

dash of olive oil

2 cloves garlic, crushed

½ red pepper, chopped

½ yellow pepper, chopped

½ orange pepper, chopped

large handful fresh organic broccoli
  (enough for 2)

1 wax free lemon

black pepper

mixed herbs

2 tbsp capers

Instructions:

Lightly brush both pieces of the Monkfish with olive oil. Cut two large pieces of tin foil. Place one quarter of garlic, capers and peppers on to *each* piece of foil, place a piece of Monkfish on top. Add the remaining peppers, capers and garlic to the top of each piece of Monkfish. Squeeze some lemon juice over both pieces. Add some mixed herbs and black pepper then fold tin foil to create a Cornish-type pasty.

Place the Monkfish parcels into preheated hot oven, gas mark 7 (220°C or 450°F) and cook for 20 minutes.

Steam broccoli for 5 minutes. Remove fish from foil and serve with broccoli.

Jasey's Hummus Cool Dipper

Serves 1

Ingredients:

small tub hummus

½ lemon

½ cucumber, cut into
   long strips

1 yellow pepper, cut into long strips

1 orange pepper, cut into long strips

1 carrot, cut into long strips

Instructions:

Place the tub of hummus in the middle of a round plate, squeeze some juice from the lemon over the top. Place the vegetables around the outside of the plate and serve.

The Juice Master's Steamed Cuisine

Serves 1

Ingredients:

8–12 oz piece lean organic
   boneless chicken breast

¼ cup organic butter

black pepper

1 lemon

1 clove garlic, crushed

2 cups broccoli, chopped

1 cup cauliflower, chopped

1 cup sweet potatoes, chopped

2 carrots, chopped

¼ cup flat leaf parsley

Instructions:

Preheat oven to gas mark 7 (220°C or 450°F). Spread some butter over both sides of chicken, add some black pepper, a squeeze of juice from the lemon and crushed garlic. Put seasoned chicken breast on to piece of tin foil and fold over leaving a little 'air-room' – like a Cornish pasty. Place in the oven and cook for 15–20 minutes.

Steam all the vegetables for 10–15 minutes.

Remove chicken from the foil and lift on to plate, pour the remaining juices over the top and the spread rest of butter over steamed vegetables. Add more black pepper and squeeze more lemon juice over the top. Sprinkle with parsley before serving.

The Juice Master's Master Muesli

Serves 1–2

Ingredients:

3 cups Juice Master's Master
   Muesli (see full recipe below)

soya milk

Juice Master's Master Muesli

1 cup jumbo porridge oats

¾ cup rye flakes

handful raisins and sultanas

4 dates, chopped

2 apricots, chopped

small handful sunflower seeds

small handful pumpkin seeds

4 Brazil nuts, chopped

6 almonds

¼ cup fresh berries

Instructions:

Put all ingredients for the Juice Master's Master Muesli into a large bowl, mix thoroughly. Add milk to serve.

Please note: you can replace the Juice Master's Master Muesli with either Organic Wheat Free Muesli or Amaranth muesli.

Jasey's Sultry Salmon with Mango and Asparagus Kicker

Serves 1 (large portion)

Ingredients:

8–10 oz piece salmon	dash balsamic vinegar
(preferably organic)	1 small mango, peeled, chopped
cold pressed virgin olive oil	1 lemon
4 spears asparagus	pinch of fresh mint
1 cup organic baby leaf	
spinach	

Instructions:

Brush both sides of fish with olive oil, meanwhile heat a frying pan until it is piping hot. Place the fish in the pan and cook on each side for 5 minutes.

Blanch the asparagus in boiling water for a couple of minutes, drain and set aside.

Meanwhile, place the spinach on plate and toss in some olive oil and a dash of balsamic vinegar.

Once cooked, place the fish on to the spinach leaves and lay the asparagus diagonally over the fish. Put the chopped mango around the fish, squeeze the juice from the lemon on top. Sprinkle fresh mint over the dish before serving.

Caesar Salad

Serves 1

Ingredients:

3 cups Iceberg lettuce	¼ cup Parmesan cheese, grated
¼ cup of Caesar dressing	1 medium/thick slice rye bread, toasted and diced

Instructions:

In a salad bowl toss together the lettuce leaves, Parmesan cheese, dressing and rye bread croutons.

Jasey's Tuna Salad with Fresh Pesto and Pineapple

Serves 1 (large portion)

Ingredients:

8–10 oz piece fresh tuna (preferably organic)

1½ lemons

½ cup baby leaf spinach

½ cup watercress

½ cup rocket leaves

2 capfuls balsamic vinegar

1 capful cold pressed virgin olive oil

freshly ground black pepper

½ apple, sliced

2 pineapple slices

Pesto

⅓ cup of fresh basil leaves, chopped finely

small handful pine nuts

1 clove garlic

some olive oil

Instructions:

Heat a frying pan until it's piping hot. Brush the fish with a little olive oil and squeeze some lemon juice on both sides. Place into the pre-heated pan. Cook on medium heat for about 5–7 minutes on each side.

Put the spinach, watercress and rocket leaves into salad bowl and add balsamic vinegar and olive oil. Toss everything together and add a little lemon juice and black pepper.

Make the pesto by pounding the basil leaves, pine nuts, garlic and olive oil in a pestle and mortar. If you don't have a pestle and mortar simply add everything into a cup and mix.

Before serving, put the dressed salad leaves on to plate, place fish on the top. Spoon the pesto on to fish and squeeze some more lemon juice over the dish. Arrange the apple and pineapple around the fish. Serve immediately.

Jasey's Green Power Toasted Wholegrain Sandwich

Serves 1

Ingredients:

2 thin slices of wholegrain/
   meal bread, toasted

1 ripe avocado, flesh only

½ cup alfalfa sprouts

½ cup watercress

1 green pepper, diced

¼ cucumber, sliced thickly

½ lemon

Instructions:

Spread the toasted bread with the avocado. Place alfalfa sprouts, watercress, pepper and cucumber on top of one slice of bread. Squeeze the juice from the lemon over the top. Top with the other slice of bread. Cut in half and serve.

Jasey's Funky Chicken with Buttered Broccoli and Courgettes

Serves 1 (large portion)

Ingredients:

½ courgette, sliced

2 cups broccoli

½ cup sweet potato, diced

2 heaped tbsp organic
   slightly salted butter

freshly ground black pepper

8–10 oz organic lean chicken

cold pressed virgin olive oil

1 lime

1 lemon

½ small red onion, chopped

1 capful balsamic vinegar

Instructions:

Steam the courgette, broccoli and sweet potato for about 10 minutes. Spread ½ tbsp butter over the vegetables and mix with some freshly ground black pepper.

Heat a frying pan until it's piping hot. Brush the chicken with some olive oil and add to the pre-heated pan. Squeeze the juice of half a lemon and lime into pan with chicken. Turn the chicken over immediately and lower the heat to medium, add the onion and balsamic vinegar. Cook for about 5 minutes on each side. To serve, place the chicken on a plate with the steamed vegetables. Spread the rest of the butter over chicken and vegetables and squeeze the juice from the remaining lemon and lime over the top.

The Juice Master's Hot 'n' Fishy Snack Attack

Serves 1

Ingredients:

2 wholemeal pitta breads,
   warmed
8 oz piece swordfish (or
   any fish or Quorn pieces)
some rocket leaves

some spinach leaves
½ lemon
capful olive oil
1 large avocado, flesh only

Instructions:

Heat some olive oil in a frying pan until hot, place in the swordfish (or Quorn), cook for 5–6 minutes on each side.

Put the rocket and spinach leaves in small bowl, squeeze the juice from the lemon and add in the olive oil.

Split the pitta breads in half and spread the insides with the avocado. Cut the fish into pieces and stuff inside the pitta breads together with the dressed salad leaves. You can add some more lemon juice or some ready made green pesto if it's too dry.

Jasey's Cod 'n' Chips

Serves 1–2

Ingredients:

2 medium sweet potatoes,
   sliced lengthways

olive oil

1 small red onion, chopped

handful mixed herbs (flat-
   leaf parsley, thyme and
   basil) finely chopped

1 clove garlic, chopped

freshly ground black pepper

1½ cups runner beans

10–14 oz cod steak

1 lemon

some butter

handful of pine nuts

Instructions:

Preheat oven to Gas Mark 7 (220°C or 425°F). Put a piece of greaseproof paper in baking tray and rub over with some olive oil. Brush sweet potatoes with some olive oil, place in the baking tray together with the onion, garlic, black pepper, pine nuts and half the herbs. Bake in middle of oven. After 15 minutes, turn over the potatoes, add in the runner beans and pour over some more olive oil. Next nestle the fish in with beans and add the rest of the herbs and a dash of lemon juice. Lightly place some tin foil over the baking tray and cook for another 15 minutes. To serve, place the cod and potato herb mixture on a plate, add more lemon juice and knob of butter.

Jasey's Quick 'n' Easy Tuna, Mayo Salad

Serves 1–2

Ingredients:

1½ 200g tins tuna steak in
   sunflower oil, drained

½ cup organic mayonnaise

1 lemon

1 yellow pepper, chopped

2 yellow or red tomatoes, sliced

½ cup cucumber, chopped

some olive oil

1 cup baby leaf spinach

½ cup alfalfa sprouts

1 carrot, grated

2 capfuls balsamic vinegar

freshly ground black pepper

Instructions:

Place tuna into a small bowl. Add mayonnaise, squeeze in half lemon and mix well together. Add in the spinach leaves, alfalfa sprouts, carrots, pepper, tomatoes and cucumber. Dress the salad with some olive oil, balsamic vinegar, the juice from the remaining lemon. Toss all the ingredients together with some freshly ground black pepper.

Jasey's Lord Sandwich

Serves 1

Ingredients:

2 slices German rye bread, toasted

1 ripe avocado, flesh only

1 cup mixed baby leaf, spinach and rocket leaves

¼ cup chopped spring onion

some organic mayonnaise

1 thin fillet lean organic chicken breast, cooked

freshly ground black pepper

½ lemon

Instructions:

Spread the toasted rye bread with the avocado flesh. Add a dash of lemon juice to each side. Place the spinach and rocket on one slice of bread and add the spring onion. Spread some mayonnaise over the chicken and place on top of the vegetables. Add black pepper and the juice from the remaining lemon. Top with the other slice of bread. Cut in half before serving.

Jasey's Stir Fried Fish and Veggie Special

Serves 1–2

Ingredients:

8–10 oz swordfish, diced

4 capfuls cold pressed
   virgin olive oil

1 lemon

2 capfuls balsamic vinegar

½ cup broccoli, chopped

½ cup courgette, sliced
   lengthwise

½ cup mange-tout

1 carrot, sliced lengthwise

½ cup red onion, diced

1 cup of red, orange and yellow
   peppers, chopped

¼ cup fennel, chopped

½ cup mixed herbs (thyme,
   basil and flat-leaf parsley)

Instructions:

Heat a pan until it's piping hot. Brush the fish pieces with some oil and place into the pan, add remaining olive oil into pan together with the juice of half a lemon and balsamic vinegar. Add the rest of ingredients and keep turning with spatula. Turn heat down a little and keep frying for about 8–10 minutes. Squeeze the juice from the remaining lemon and serve.

Stuffed Pepper Supreme with Pesto

Serves 1–2

Ingredients:

1 cup baby spinach leaves

1 apple, chopped

1 cup alfalfa sprouts

½ cup raisins

1 ripe avocado, flesh only,
   diced

2 tsp sunflower seeds

1 lemon

1 yellow pepper, top removed
   and deseeded

1 orange pepper, top removed
   and deseeded

Pesto

⅓ cup fresh basil leaves   small handful pine nuts

1 clove garlic   some olive oil

Instructions:

Put spinach, apple, sprouts, raisins, avocado and sunflower seeds into bowl.

Make the pesto by pounding the basil leaves, garlic, pine nuts, and olive oil in a pestle and mortar. If you don't have a pestle and mortar simply add everything into a cup and mix.

Add pesto to bowl containing the spinach mixture, squeeze lemon over the top, mix thoroughly and stuff into each of the peppers.

Jasey's Lip Licking Lemon Chicken with Broccoli Chaser (*if veggie replace with Quorn fillet*)

Serves 1

Ingredients:

8–10 oz of organic filleted   freshly ground black pepper

   chicken breast   2 cups broccoli

1 lemon   small knob of organic unsalted

small handful mixed herbs   or lightly salted butter

Instructions:

Pre-heat the oven to a medium heat. Place chicken on piece of tin foil, squeeze half of lemon on both sides and then add mixed herbs and freshly ground pepper. Fold tin foil to cover all of the chicken and place in oven for 20–25 minutes.

Meanwhile, steam the broccoli for about 10 minutes, or until just still crunchy.

Once cooked, remove chicken from foil and place on to hot plate. Add the broccoli and spread knob of butter over. Squeeze rest of lemon over the lot.

Jasey's Honey-glazed Salmon, Papaya and Rocket Salad

Serves 1

Ingredients:

8–10 oz salmon fillets	3 yellow cherry tomatoes, halved
some cold pressed virgin	3 red cherry tomatoes, halved
olive oil	1 lemon
some manuka active honey	½ cup spring onion, diced
some balsamic vinegar	½ papaya, diced
2 cups rocket leaves	

Instructions:

Heat a frying pan until it's piping hot. Brush the fish with some olive oil, balsamic vinegar and honey and add to the pan, brown for about 10 seconds on both sides and lower the heat to medium. Continue cooking for 5 minutes on each side. Turn the heat up and squeeze the juice from the lemon to finish off.

Meanwhile, place the rocket leaves and spring onions in the centre of a plate. Arrange the tomatoes in alternate colours around the rocket. Drizzle some olive oil and balsamic vinegar on top of the rocket leaves. Brush some honey on the papaya chunks and arrange over the top of the rocket.

To serve, place the fish on to the salad leaves and lightly brush with honey.

Jasey's Tuna Mayo and Rye Bread Snack Attack

Serves 1

Ingredients:

200g tuna steak canned in	½ lemon
water or sunflower oil,	¼ cup organic mayonnaise
drained	freshly ground black pepper
½ ripe large avocado, flesh only	2 slices German rye bread, toasted

236

Instructions:

Place the tuna and avocado into a bowl, squeeze the juice from the lemon and add the mayonnaise and black pepper. Mix thoroughly and spread on to each slice of rye bread. Serve this with a cup of peppermint tea with small spoonful of Manuka honey!

Jasey's Fish Kebabs with Pineapple and Steamed Veggies

Serves 1

Ingredients:

10 oz swordfish steak	⅓ small pineapple, peeled and cubed
some olive oil	¼ cup slightly salted organic butter
1 lemon	freshly ground black pepper
2 cups broccoli	some balsamic vinegar
4 asparagus spears	

Instructions:

Pre-heat a grill to its highest setting. Brush the fish lightly with olive oil and balsamic vinegar and place on tray in middle part of the grill. Cook for 3 minutes on each side and lower the heat to medium. Squeeze the juice of the lemon on to the fish and cook for a couple of minutes. Remove and cut fish into cubes.

Steam the broccoli for 8–10 minutes, and the asparagus for 2 minutes.

To make the kebabs, thread cubes of pineapple and fish alternately on to a skewer. You should end up with three skewers of kebabs. Place skewers underneath a hot grill for 2 minutes turning them over half way through.

To serve, place the broccoli and asparagus on plate, spread butter over and add some ground pepper. Place the skewers over veggies and serve.

Jasey's Quick 'n' Easy Hot Pittas and Dip

Serves 1

Ingredients:

1 tub hummus

½ ripe avocado, flesh only, chopped

½ cup spring onion, chopped

1 lemon

2 wholemeal pitta breads, toasted, cut into strips

Instructions:

Put the hummus on a plate and mix in the avocado, spring onion and squeeze the juice from the lemon over the top. Serve with pitta strips.

Hot 'n' Cold Veggie Delight

Serves 1–2

Ingredients:

10 oz Quorn pieces

some olive oil

some balsamic vinegar

1 cup broccoli, chopped

½ cup mange-tout, chopped

½ cup red cabbage, grated

2 carrots, grate one and slice the other lengthways

1 cup baby spinach

½ cup rocket

knob of organic butter

freshly ground black pepper

1 lemon

Instructions:

Brush the Quorn pieces with some olive oil and balsamic vinegar. Heat a frying pan until it's piping hot. Add in the Quorn pieces, stirring occasionally. Lower the heat to medium.

Add the broccoli, mange-tout, ¼ of the red cabbage and the sliced carrot to pan. Add some more oil and balsamic vinegar, stirring the mixture occasionally. Continue cooking for about 8 minutes.

Place the spinach and rocket leaves on a plate and drizzle some olive oil and balsamic vinegar over the top.

To serve, place the Quorn and vegetable mixture on top of the salad leaves. Top with butter. Add the remaining red cabbage and carrot. Squeeze the juice from the lemon over the top and finish off with some black pepper. If this dish is too dry you can add some green pesto.

Pitta Bread Salad

Serves 1–2

Ingredients:

1 cup Cos lettuce

1 large tomato, diced

2 inch cucumber, cubed

1 spring onion, diced

½ small red onion, diced

1 red, yellow or green
    pepper, diced

1 tbsp fresh parsley, roughly
    chopped

½ tbsp fresh mint, chopped

1 wholemeal pitta bread,
    toasted, cut into squares

Lemon dressing

1 fl oz olive oil

zest of ¼ lemon

1 tbsp lemon juice

freshly ground black pepper

Instructions:

Combine the salad vegetables and chopped herbs in a large salad bowl. Toss to mix. In separate bowl combine the ingredients for dressing, whisk and season with black pepper. Spoon the dressing over the salad leaves and toss again. Scatter the pitta bread over the top and toss before serving.

Fresh Tuna with Cracked Pepper and Coriander with Rocket Salad

Serves 1

Ingredients:

8–10 oz tuna steak

some olive oil

½ tbsp black peppercorns,
   coarsely crushed

½ tbsp coriander seeds,
   coarsely crushed

½ tbsp balsamic vinegar

2 tbsp olive oil

1 cup rocket leaves

6 cherry tomatoes, halved

pepper to season

fresh chives, roughly chopped

Instructions:

Brush the tuna with olive oil. Mix the crushed peppercorns and coriander and roll the tuna in the mixture until thoroughly coated. Wrap up tightly in foil.

Heat a heavy cast-iron pan until it's piping hot. Lay the foil-wrapped tuna in the pan and cook for 10 minutes, turning it every minute or so – make sure that each side gets cooked. Take the tuna out of pan and leave to cool.

Whisk balsamic vinegar with olive oil to make the dressing and add pinch of pepper to taste.

Toss the rocket leaves and tomatoes in the dressing and arrange on plate. Unwrap tuna, slice and lay it on top of salad. Scatter chopped chives and serve immediately.

Snacks

Avocado and Sardines

Ingredients:

One de-stoned avocado

1 tin sardines (95g boneless in sunflower oil)

½ lemon

Instructions:

Place the sardines and avocado in a small bowl. Squeeze on the lemon juice, mix together and serve.

JM's Snack Attack

Ingredients:

1 slice rye bread

½ ripe avocado

½ cup alfalfa sprouts

½ lime

Instructions:

Toast the rye bread and spread on the avocado. Place the alfalfa sprouts on top and squeeze on lime juice to garnish.

JM's Small Cucumber Dipper

Ingredients:

⅓ cucumber

Small tub ready-made hummus

½ lemon

Instructions:

Cut the cucumber into lengthway slices. Squeeze the lemon into the hummus. Dip slices into the hummus and eat.

You can easily change the above recipe to include any other vegetables – peppers, carrots and celery also taste great.

JM's Wholemeal Pitta Snack

Ingredients:

1 wholemeal pitta bread

1 ready-made tub of guacamole OR hummus

Instructions:

Toast pitta bread and cut into strips. Then dunk into chosen dip and eat.

JM's Sun-dried Tomatoes and Olives

Ingredients:

Handful of olives (any kind, but black pitted go best)

Small handful of sun-dried tomatoes

Instructions:

Mix ingredients together and serve.

Tinned Fish Snack

Ingredients:

1 95g tin sardines OR tuna

½ lemon

Instructions:

Open the tin and drain the oil from the fish. Squeeze the lemon juice over the fish and serve immediately.

Organic Rye Crackers

Ingredients:

2 wholemeal rye crackers

½ avocado

Instructions:

Spread avocado over the rye crackers and serve. As an alternative, organic butter or another natural topping of your choice can be just as tasty.

Oat Cakes

Ingredients:

1 or 2 oat cakes (make sure you get a good source – without
   sugar and too many addictives)

½ avocado OR a knob of organic butter

A small serving of the vegetable of your choice e.g ⅓ cucumber
   OR 1 tomato.

Instructions:

Spread the avocado or butter on the oat cakes. Add the vegetable of your choice – cucumber, spring onion and tomatoes work well. Serve.

Soups

As a snack, soup is always a nice idea – especially on a cold winter's day. Choose a fresh soup from a range like the New Covent Garden Food Company. If you want bread with it, have 1 slice of wholemeal bread with a little organic butter. Avoid this side serving of bread if you can help it though.

Organic Boiled Eggs

Boiled eggs make a great little snack. Hard boiled eggs take twelve minutes to cook, simmering in a saucepan of lightly salted water. You can mix them in a bowl with chopped peppers, cucumber or celery – or simply eat them as they are. Make sure you don't overdo it and only have the one egg for a snack.

Juicy Snack

One of the best options to curb hunger is to make a quick juice. Fat helps to regulate the appetite, so it's a good idea to mix an avocado in with a veggie juice or put some nuts in with a fruit juice.

Dried Fruits and Nuts

Dried fruits can be high in sugar and not always the best thing to have when trying to lose weight. However, this doesn't mean that you should avoid all dried fruits; just make sure you go easy on them. Dried fruits are very 'moreish', so it's important not to gorge yourself on them as you perhaps would with sweets or biscuits. Keep to one conservative handful for a snack portion size. This same principle applies to natural nuts. The best dried fruits to have are raisins, unsulphured apricots and figs. For a treat you cannot beat dried mango – it's heaven!

Organic Date and Apricot Slices (Wheat free)

Many will be glad to see these on the menu. They aren't the ideal snack, but every now and then they are OK. They are like flapjacks, only healthier. I recommend the brand made by the Village Bakery – these are available from Sainsbury's. Please be careful not to overdo it – a snack portion is 'just the one'; any more would constitute a small meal.

The Best Snack of All

The best snack is always going to be a piece of low sugar fruit or some nuts. You cannot beat the humble organic apple to help raise sugar levels (gradually) and supply the body with easy to digest nutrients. See below for some suggestions of my favourite fruits for snacks:

Acceptable fruit chart

Apples	Apricots
Satsumas	Pears
Kiwis	Grapefruits
Avocados	Pumpkins
Tomatoes	Cantaloupes
Berries	Cherries
Oranges	Plums
Limes	Mangos
Honeydews	Peaches
Tangerines	Dried apricots

appendix d

the 'new you' shopping list

Tips for stocking up at home

What To Keep In Your Cupboard

As you have seen from the 21 day plan, the 'New You' plan for life focuses on the consumption of fresh natural produce – and I recommend that the majority of your intake is made up of natural goods. However, it is not *all* you will be eating – so here are some suggestions of the non-fresh foods you should keep in the house.

Pasta (wholemeal or wheat free)

Rice (whole grain)

Rye bread

Wheat free organic muesli

Organic rye flakes

Organic jumbo porridge oats

Organic oat cakes

Dark Ryvita

Marmite (OK on a slice of rye bread)

Manuka active honey (available at Sainsbury's)

Pesto (green or red)

Sun-dried tomatoes

Capers

Tins of sardines, tuna and mackerel (keep plenty in, these are great as a quick snack with lemon or lime juice)

Soya milk

Various teas – peppermint, camomile, lemon & ginger and so on

Cold pressed virgin olive oil

White balsamic vinegar

Dark balsamic vinegar

Nuts (natural – never roasted or salted)

Cinnamon

Nutmeg

Mixed herbs

Ginger spice

Black pepper (freshly ground)

In The Freezer

When you freeze fruits and vegetables you only lose about 5% of the nutrient content, so it's always a good idea to keep a good stock of them in – just in case you cannot buy fresh.

Frozen fruits – great for making quick smoothies, most good supermarkets sell various bags of frozen fruits. You can also cut some fresh fruit and freeze it yourself as an alternative.

Frozen vegetables – frozen veggies can come in very handy, especially if you've missed the supermarket or haven't had the time. Frozen is often not as good as fresh, but it still contains plenty of wonderful nutrients. You can also juice vegetables straight from frozen, which is not only handy, but also makes the most wonderful-tasting, refreshing juice.

Quorn Fillets (if veggie), **Fish and Chicken**. Once again fresh is always best, but when needs must these additions to your freezer can come in very handy. Prawns are particularly good to have in as they mix well with a quick and easy stir fry.

Quick Fix Meals

Your best bet in an emergency is to keep in stock a frozen stir fry. It's not the best choice of meal in the whole world, as the rice will often be white – but white rice isn't as bad as white flour, and a meal like this could make the difference between you going for a takeaway and actually realising you've got something pretty healthy in. The idea is not to get 'caught short'. That's why it's good to have a stock of foods in the house, which will mean you don't have to turn to the land of the takeaways on those nights when you feel too tired for 'proper' cooking.

One other addition to your home, and a Juice Master favourite:

Stay Fresh For Longer Bags

These are an amazing invention. They are food bags which have the ability to keep your fruits and veg super fresh for weeks in the fridge! This means you can cut up some fruit and veg ready for a juice recipe, put it into a Stay Fresh For Longer Bag and simply juice in the morning. You could do this with the whole week's recipes – so that you can just wake up, juice and go! Cutting as you juice is generally better, as the produce will be dew-fresh, but if you don't have the time then this is the next best thing. To see where you can get these wonder bags go to www.thejuicemaster.com.

appendix e

sources of nutrients

Vitamins	Functions	Sources in the diet
Vitamin A	Needed for vision in dim light; for maintenance of skin and mucous membranes (such as inside your mouth and nose), and growth.	Milk, fortified margarines, butter, cheese, egg yolk, liver, fatty fish, fish liver oils, carrots, tomatoes, spinach, red peppers, broccoli.
Vitamin D	Helps the absorption of calcium and phosphate from food. Essential for development and maintenance of strong bones and teeth.	Fortified margarines and fat spreads, fatty fish, egg yolk, fortified breakfast cereals – and sunshine!
Vitamin E	Protects cell membranes from damage.	Vegetable oils, nuts and cereals.
Vitamin K	Needed for blood clotting.	Spinach, broccoli, kale, cabbage, Brussel sprouts and dried seaweed. This vitamin is also made by bacteria in the gut.
Vitamin C	Needed to make collagen which is used in the structure of connective tissue and bone. Helps wound healing and iron absorption.	Citrus fruits, strawberries, kiwi fruit, guava, berries, green pepper, broccoli, cabbage, kale. Also found in potatoes.
Thiamin (Vitamin B1)	Involved in the release of energy from carbohydrate. It is important for the brain and nerves which use glucose for their energy needs.	Yeast, yeast extracts, pork, wholegrain cereals (brown rice, wholemeal bread), nuts and pulses green vegetables, fortified breakfast cereals.
Riboflavin (Vitamin B2)	Involved in energy release – especially from fat and protein.	Yeast, yeast extracts, liver, milk, cheese, yogurt, green vegetables, and fortified cereals.
Niacin	Involved in the release of energy from food.	Yeast extracts, liver, beef, pork, lamb, fish, fortified breakfast cereals, wholegrain cereals.
Vitamin B12	Necessary for the creation of healthy blood cells and nerve fibres.	Offal and meat, eggs, milk and fortified breakfast cereals. Almost no plant foods contain B12.

Vitamins	Functions	Sources in the diet
Pyridoxine (Vitamin B6)	Needed to help make healthy blood.	Pork, beef, lamb, bananas, nuts, pulses, fortified breakfast cereals and wholegrain cereals.
Folate	Needed for the development of healthy blood cells. Reduces the risk of neural tube defects in babies.	Liver, yeast extracts, oranges, dark green vegetables and fortified breakfast cereals.
Biotin	Needed in the production of many different enzymes in the body.	Offal, yeast, nuts, pulses, wholegrain cereals and eggs.
Pantothenic acid	Needed to help release energy in the body.	Offal, yeast, eggs, nuts, pork, lamb, beef and green vegetables

Minerals	Functions	Sources in the diet
Calcium	Needed for the development and maintenance of strong bones and teeth. Helps blood to clot and aids nerve function.	Milk, cheese, yogurt, fromage frais, canned fish with bones, green leafy vegetables, pulses, white and brown flour and bread, tap water in hard water areas.
Sodium	Helps in the regulation of the water content in the body. Needed for nerve function.	Salt, ham, bacon, smoked foods, cheese, yeast extracts, breads, salted nuts, crisps.
Potassium	Needed for proper functioning of body cells, muscles and nerves.	Present in most foods except sugars, fats and oils.
Magnesium	Needed to help release energy in the body. Needed for healthy development of the skeleton, proper function of the muscles, and making protein.	Green vegetables, meats, pulses, wholegrain cereals and nuts.
Phosphorus	An essential component of all cells and present in bones and teeth.	Milk, cheese, meat, fish, eggs, nuts, cereals, fruits and vegetables.
Iron	Needed in the formation of haemoglobin to make healthy red blood cells.	Red meat, offal, cereals, bread, green leafy vegetables, fortified breakfast cereals, dried fruit, nuts and seeds.
Zinc	Essential for growth, sexual maturation and the immune system.	Milk, cheese, red meat, eggs and fish, shellfish, chicken, wholegrain cereals, green leafy vegetables and pulses.
Iodine	Needed in the formation of thyroid hormones.	Milk, seafood, seaweed. Iodised salt.
Fluoride	Makes teeth more resistant to decay.	Fluoridated water, tea, fish and toothpaste.
Selenium	Protects cell membranes against damage.	Cereals, meat, fish, offal, cheese, vegetables and eggs.

Macronutrients	Functions	Sources in the diet
Protein	Needed for growth and repair of body tissues. Can also be used to provide energy. Protein is made up of amino acids. Amino acids can be divided into two types – *indispensable* (which cannot be made in the body and have to be supplied by foods) and *dispensable* (which can be made in the body). Proportions of indispensable and dispensable amino acids vary in different foods. Animal sources contain a higher proportion of indispensable amino acids compared to vegetable sources.	Beef, lamb, pork, duck, fish, shellfish, chicken, eggs, nuts, pulses, beans, tofu, cheese, offal, Quorn, textured vegetable protein.
Fat	Provides a concentrated source of energy to the body. Fat helps the absorption of fat-soluble vitamins A, D, E and K and is used for their transportation throughout the blood. It helps maintain healthy skin and hair. Essential fatty acids help to ensure proper growth and development in infants and can also reduce the risk of heart disease. Fat is made up of three different types: saturated, monounsaturated and polyunsaturated fats. Most fats contain all three types, but in varying proportions. Saturated fats can lead to high levels of *bad* cholesterol, which can clog up arteries and may eventually lead to heart disease. Monounsaturated fats help raise the levels of *good* cholesterol. Some polyunsaturated fats are called essential fats because they can't be made in the body and have to be obtained from the diet; omega-3 fats can help reduce the tendency for blood to clot, while omega-6 fats are essential for maintaining the structure and function of body tissues. Eating less saturated fats and more essential fats can help decrease the risk of developing heart disease.	Saturated fats: animal fats, milk, cheese, butter. Monounsaturated fats: nuts, olive oil, peanut butter, avocados. Polyunsaturated fats: plants and fish. Omega-3 fats: oily fish such as mackerel, sardines, salmon and pilchards. Omega-6 fats: vegetable seeds and polyunsaturated margarines.
Carbohydrate	There are two types of carbohydrates found in food – complex carbohydrates (starches and fibre) and simple carbohydrates (sugars). Starches and sugars provide energy to the body. Simple sugars are easily digested to glucose and enter the bloodstream shortly after eating. This can cause a rapid rise in blood sugar levels. If blood sugar levels rise too high, insulin is released to clear out the excess. Complex carbohydrates are digested more slowly than simple sugars and release glucose at a slower rate, resulting in a steadier level of blood sugar. There are two types of fibre – insoluble fibre which helps to maintain a healthy gut and soluble fibre which helps to reduce blood cholesterol.	Starches: potatoes, bread, rice, pasta, grains. Naturally occuring sugars: milk, fruits, vegetables. Processed sugars: jam, sweets, soft drinks, table sugar. Soluble fibre: fruits, vegetables, oats, pulses, beans.

appendix f

10 FAQs (Frequently Asked Questions) about boosting your metabolism

1. What is metabolism and why is it important?

Think of your metabolism as the engine in your body. It's like a little furnace, burning away all day and night, fuelled both by the food you eat and the fat you have within your body. The more muscle you have, the more fuel your engine will need to tick over. Because of genetics, some women burn fat faster than others. But age, weight, diet and exercise habits also play a role. As we grow older, our metabolisms slow down, mainly because we are losing five or six pounds of muscle each decade starting in the mid-20s. That means we might all be burning 100 fewer calories a day at 35 than at 25, despite doing nothing differently. But there are easy things you can do to keep your metabolism burning high, or stoke it up after it's become sluggish. Make sure you get plenty of sleep – it helps keep your metabolism running well. In a recent study, people who got four hours of sleep or less a night had more difficulty processing carbohydrates. When you're exhausted, your body lacks the energy to do its normal day-to-day functions, which include burning calories, so your metabolism is automatically lowered.

2. What's the best way to boost my metabolism?

The only way to directly build your metabolic rate (think of it like the turnover rate of your engine) is to build muscle, which means weight training! When most people want to lose weight, as well as going on a diet they try doing some cardio workouts – like going to aerobics classes, running on a treadmill or riding an exercise bike. That's fine... to burn some calories. But to actually increase the rate at which your body burns fat, then you have to have more muscle. For every pound of muscle gained, you burn an extra 70 calories per hour, just at rest!

3. What about eating lots of protein – doesn't that boost metabolism?

Eating more protein will not necessarily result in muscle growth. Your body can only use a certain amount of protein each day; after that your body will store the excess as fat. Consuming 40–50 grams of protein a day is sufficient for muscle growth and tissue repair. So eat lean proteins like eggs, lean beef, chicken and fish, and combine them with colourful carbohydrates like fruits and veggies (high in natural enzymes, vitamins and minerals). Research shows that getting the right amount of protein *can* boost your metabolism, causing you to burn an extra 150 to 200 calories a day. That's because protein is made up of amino acids, which are harder for your body to break down than fat and carbs, so you burn more calories in processing them.

4. What about eating a diet of 'negative calorie' foods?

'Negative calories' is a new phrase that's just flown in from the States, where some experts reckon that certain foods take more calories to digest than the calories the foods actually contain. So, a 25 calorie piece of broccoli (100 grams) requires 80 calories to digest, resulting in a net loss of 55 calories from the body fat! Thus, the more you eat, the more you lose weight!! It all sounds a little too good to be true, doesn't it? But coincidentally, the so-called 'negative calorie' foods are all good for you – so eat away! They include the following: asparagus, beets, broccoli, cabbage, carrots, cauliflower, celery, cucumbers, garlic, lettuce, onions, spinach, turnip, courgettes, apples, cranberries, grapefruit, lemons, mangos, oranges, pineapple, raspberries, strawberries and tangerines!

5. Can drinking ice cold water boost your metabolic rate?

The negative calorie people also say that drinking cold water causes you to burn calories simply to heat up your body again. Others say drinking water at room temperature is better for you, as the water is more quickly absorbed by the body. Water is essential for all bodily functions and dehydration can lead to fatigue, edginess and an inability to concentrate. Plus, some experts believe that a dehydrated body is unable to burn fat quickly. Aim for the recommended eight tall glasses of water a day.

6. I've heard that spicy foods can speed up your metabolism. True?

Certain spices can apparently give your weight loss an added boost – though I suspect that they would make a microscopic difference, so don't splurge out on a chicken jalfrezi tonight just because it is spicy! Certain experts say that ginger, cloves, cayenne, coriander, bay leaves and dry mustard have all demonstrated a 'thermogenic' or fat-burning effect, thus raising metabolism. Capsaicin, a compound found in certain spices and peppers, temporarily stimulates your body to release more stress hormones such as adrenalin, speeding up your metabolism and increasing your ability to burn calories. Whether it is true or not, spicy foods will make you drink more water – which is good!

7. What's all this about omega-3 oils helping you to lose weight?

Omega-3 oils are the ones that are very good for you – and researchers are still discovering their disease-prevention properties. Dieticians reckon that these are fats you should be eating *even* if you want to lose weight – and they may even help boost the metabolism. You'll get the cold fish oils from salmon, herring, mackerel, sardines and tuna (though canned tuna is not a good source of omega-3 fats). Sample linseed oil too, either as a supplement in pill form or mixed into your salad dressings. Dieticians in the USA are beginning to get very excited about this oil – as well as boosting the metabolism, it is thought to be able to lower cholesterol, banish arthritis and migraines, and can also help control asthma. It will make you feel full and satisfied after a meal.

8. Does chewing gum keep your metabolism going?

After exhaustive research, I have found that chewing gum apparently burns about 11 calories an hour. I suppose that's better than nothing, if you are absolutely